I0475967

Central Pain Syndrome

Chronic, Confounding Pain Such As That Of Fibromyalgia

By The Same Author

SNA: Theory and Practice
Reengineering IBM Networks
Integrating TCP/IP i-nets with IBM Data Centers
Corporate Portals Empowered with XML and Web Services
Web Services: Theory and Practice

Popes and the Tale of Their Names
The Next Pope
The Next Pope 2011
The Last 9 Conclaves
The Last 10 Conclaves: 2013 to 1903
The Election of the 2013 Pope
Pope Names for the 2013 Conclave
Pope John XXIII: 101 Facts & Trivia
Popes: 101 Facts & Trivia
Pope Francis' U.S. Visit -- 2015

Comet ISON, C/2012 S1 (ISON)
Comet ISON, C/2012 S1 (ISON) Quick Reference
Comet ISON for Kids
Comets: 101 Facts & Trivia

Devanee's Book of Dwarf Planets
Matthew's Book of 4 Vesta the Would be Planet

Orgasms: 101 Facts & Trivia

Teischan's ABC Book of Great Artists
A Pup is NOT a Toy

Brain Meditation – For True Productivity & Serenity
Quick Guide to Brain Meditation

All available from Amazon (worldwide).

Central Pain Syndrome

Chronic, Confounding Pain Such As That Of Fibromyalgia

Anura Guruge

Edition One
April 2017

WOWNH LLC
New Hampshire
USA
www.wownh.com

Copyright © 2017, Anura Gurugé.
All Rights Reserved.

No part of this book may be reproduced, stored in a retrieval system, or transmitted by any means without the written permission of the author.

First published by WOWNH LLC in April 2017.

ISBN-10: 1544186622
ISBN-13: 978-1544186627

Printed in the United States of America

This book is printed on acid-free paper.

PHOTOGRAPHIC CREDITS: All of the images used in this book, including that on the cover, are public domain material (from the likes of Wikipedia) – with attribution included where appropriate.

To
All Those Affected,
Directly or Indirectly,
by Central Pain Syndrome
or Fibromyalgia

CONTENTS

Chapters 1 to 6 contain, at the end, a one-page
'*Takeaways*' section that *summarizes*
the *key points* from that chapter.

Refer to index for ***Fibromyalgia*** references.

PREFACE

I wrote this book because I was unable to find a *self-help guide* to **Central Pain Syndrome (CPS)** when I went looking for one, on Amazon, in early 2016. The only books I was able to locate were for medical professionals rather than for those actually living with CPS.

I do not have CPS and neither am I a doctor. I have, however, been living with CPS and its myriad quirks, frustrations and setbacks since 2011. CPS has altered and redefined my life; alas, not for the better.

My wife has CPS. It was I, who four years ago, after extensive Web research, determined that this had to be what it was. When I raised it with her then Pain Doctor he grudgingly admitted that it was so, though he had never told us so. During the last 5 years, and in well over 40 visits with my wife to various doctors and other healthcare professionals, I have only had one other 'doctor' mention CPS – and that too at my instigation. In my experience 'doctors' do not like to talk about CPS. They prefer to call it *fibromyalgia* though many of them should know better!

My wife suffered a spinal injury in 2006, working as a Licensed Nursing Assistant (LNA) at a nursing home, in the process of moving an elderly patient. It was serious enough for her to be deemed permanently disabled. She finally decided, in early 2011, to undergo spinal fusion surgery; her mobility by then had been severely compromised. Following the initial month of intense pain, the surgery appeared to have been a success. So much so that six-months later, she and her pain doctor felt that it was appropriate to scale back her pain medication – which had included opioids. Six weeks later, as I like to describe it: *'all hell broke loose'*! She started having pains here, there and everywhere. In my opinion that was the start of her CPS. Others, including my wife, might not agree.

Yes, she was diagnosed with fibromyalgia. She was 'treated' for fibromyalgia. Over the years, she has been on numerous medications and has had dozens of injections, epidural, facet joint, etc. There has also been acupuncture, physical therapy and more appointments than I care to recall. She has had TENS units and of late is a near daily user of the Aleve wireless unit (which I obtained for her from Walmart for $50). So, I have hands-on experience of much of what I talk about in this book.

CPS sucks. I know that. I live with that, *daily*. So, I can empathize.

CPS has redefined my life and I don't have CPS (at least not as yet). So, I wrote this book as much for those in my shoes as for those in my wife's. As far as I am concerned we, '*the affected*', are all in the same boat.

This is meant to be a **self-help book** – not a medical treatise. I am fairly certain that there is nothing in this book that can hurt YOU. Anything that I talk about, which has the potential to harm, *if done legally*, requires a prescription from or involvement of a doctor or a licensed medical professional. *{SMILE}* So just reading this book can only help YOU and those around you. I fail to see how it can hinder.

CPS is NOT easy to contend with. That doctors, at least in the U.S., appear to be reluctant to confront CPS, head-on, as they should, does not help matters. CPS, in my opinion, is a **taboo** condition. I am convinced that CPS is far more widespread than even the '*few million*' currently believed to be CPS sufferers. I am sure that there are many who have CPS, but do not have a clue they have a condition to do with their central nervous system rather than a real injury/inflammation somewhere else. I really hope we can, together, increase awareness of CPS – or maybe '*Central Sensitization*', an even broader categorization. CPS a subset of it.

CPS, in my opinion, is something you really have to get *your mind around*. When you have pain, burning, numbness, or discomfort, that seems to be so specific and so pressing, it is hard to accept the pain might, in reality, be due to a 'short circuit' in the central nervous system. That is hard to process, acknowledge and accept. The pain and discomfort is always so specific. So definite. The problem being that none of us have the experience to appreciate pain arising as a result of a central nervous system *disorder*. We are so conditioned to associate pain with an injury, inflammation or infection. But, alas, that is not so with CPS. You have to, at some point, come to terms with CPS. In order to do so, you have to understand what CPS is all about. *Hence, this book.*

In my opinion it helps to know as much as you can about CPS. The more you know the better you can be about understanding what is happening *to you* and what options you have. That was another reason for this book. As my pricing should indicate, I did not write this book in the hope of making any money. Given the 'fixed costs' involved (and imposed by the likes of Amazon), which are well outside of my control, both the print and eBook are being marketed altruistically. {SMILE}

I really hope this books helps you. In my experience those affected by CPS need all the help they can get. I have been surprised and frustrated as to how little attention there is to CPS. It is an overlooked and ignored condition. Yes, many in 'the profession' will admit that it, like fibromyalgia, is not well understood. Much of that has to be attributed to insufficient study and research – and that eventually has to do with inadequate funding.

I, however, detect a shift in fortunes. Chronic pain, epidemic in scope, has got to the point that it is taking a significant, hard-to-ignore toll on worldwide economies. CPS falls squarely within the bounds of chronic pain. As such I am hoping the tide will soon start to change. There are some new drugs awaiting clinical trials. They more closely mimic the body's own natural pain reducing 'chemicals' than anything currently available. They hold some real promise and could revolutionize pain treatment. But, they are unlikely to be available in the U.S. till well past the year 2021. So, we need to somehow get through till then – or beyond.

I should explain at this juncture that I, among other things, was a professional, technical writer for over 30-years. I have an extensive body of printed work, books and publications, covering diverse subjects from computer networking to popes. If I can research it, I can write about it. That is how this book, like so many of my others, came to be. I should also mention that I have been interested in the workings of the brain ever since I was a teenager. I am a proponent of a very concentrated form of meditation that I refer to as '*Brain Meditation*'. In 2016 I wrote two books about it. The brain plays a huge part in CPS. As such, I was already on a role when I started writing this book.

I wish you the very best. **We are in this together**. You can contact me at: _anu@wownh.com_. I am fairly easy to find on the Web. {SMILE}

Anura Gurugé
Lakes Region, New Hampshire,
March 2017

1.
AN OVERVIEW

Central Pain Syndrome can be all of this and more:

Pins-and-Needles **Burning** *Cutting* Tightness

Aching *Agonizing Pain* Anxiety *Fatigue*

Stiffness Confusion *Body on Fire* Muscle Spasms

Stabbing **Forgetfulness** *Freezing*

Walking Barefoot on Sharp Rocks Throbbing

Numbness Crushing **Multiple Pains**

Excruciating *Unrelenting* Nausea

Clothes Hurt/Scratch Depression

Hurts When Touched *Every Movement Hurts*

Searing *Pressing* **Bursts of Sharp Pain**

Being Cut With Razor Blades

Unimaginable Pain

Dreading being asked: "how are you?"

OTHER CHARACTERIZATIONS OF
CENTRAL PAIN SYNDROME MAY INCLUDE:

❖ *Sensitization* of the pain system
  [i.e., being more 'sensitive', or in this case, the body's pain system amplifying, over time, how it responds to the pain signals it receives].

❖ Damage to, or dysfunction of, the **Central Nervous System** (CNS).

❖ The volume control of your body's pain system being turned way up.

❖ Persistent pain from anywhere in the body.

❖ Neurological disorder, i.e., a disorder of the **nervous system**.

❖ Pain that is *not caused* by any harmful 'stimulus' to the body (i.e., injury, impact, touch or infection).

❖ Pain that originates in the central nervous system (and not in the peripheral nerves).

❖ Lifelong *neurological disease* of the *central nervous system* (i.e., a disease of the nervous system).

❖ Marked, lifestyle altering behavioral changes due to pain.

❖ Caused by a *disruption* to how the brain processes pain.

❖ Constant, never-ending, agonizing pain from all parts of the body.

❖ **Brain *out-of-control* in terms of handling pain.**

❖ Tends to affect one's arm or foot with intense pain, sometimes quite dramatically – along with possible localized swelling and changes in skin color/texture.

❖ <u>No</u> injury/inflammation to a joint/muscle causing the pain.

❖ Prolonged pain that cannot be associated with a specific injury or inflammation.

❖ *Closely related to Fibromyalgia.*

❖ Character of the pain differs widely among sufferers; probably due to the variety of potential causes.

❖ Brain gone *haywire* when it comes to dealing with *any* pain.

❖ Voluntarily, but with a sense of helplessness, forgoing once cherished activities, social interactions, hobbies and pastimes due.

CENTRAL NERVOUS SYSTEM & CENTRAL PAIN SYNDROME

All formal, medical definitions of Central Pain Syndrome (**CPS**) invariably begin by stating that it is a: *neurological condition* caused by damage to or dysfunction of the *central nervous system* (**CNS**). [Neurological = Nervous System] So, it is best to have some understanding of the central nervous system when trying to deal with CPS.

Your central nervous system consists of your brain and spinal cord. Refer to the diagrams below. Some might say brain and '*brain stem*', while others include the brain stem as an integral part of the brain.

CPS is thus caused by some kind of violation that happened to one's brain and/or spinal cord. There is **no other** injury or inflammation in another part of the body responsible for the *CPS-related pain*. There could be *other* pain, in *addition*, which will get *amplified* by CPS.

This is the *current* understanding and medical consensus when it comes to CPS. Whether you like it or not, when it comes to CPS you have to think in terms of something that has gone wrong within your brain and/or spinal cord; *nowhere else*. There is no getting around this, at least for now.

CPS, AS SUCH, HAS ALL TO DO WITH THE CENTRAL NERVOUS SYSTEM.

The '**central**' in CPS points to this connection.

The central nervous system is the body's one and only 'command and control' center. All activity to do with thought, the control of movement and 'feeling' of sensations (including pain) is handled by the central nervous system. It is what collects, processes and makes sense of all information received from other parts of the body (including the eyes and ears). It then coordinates and directs our actions based on the information it has processed.

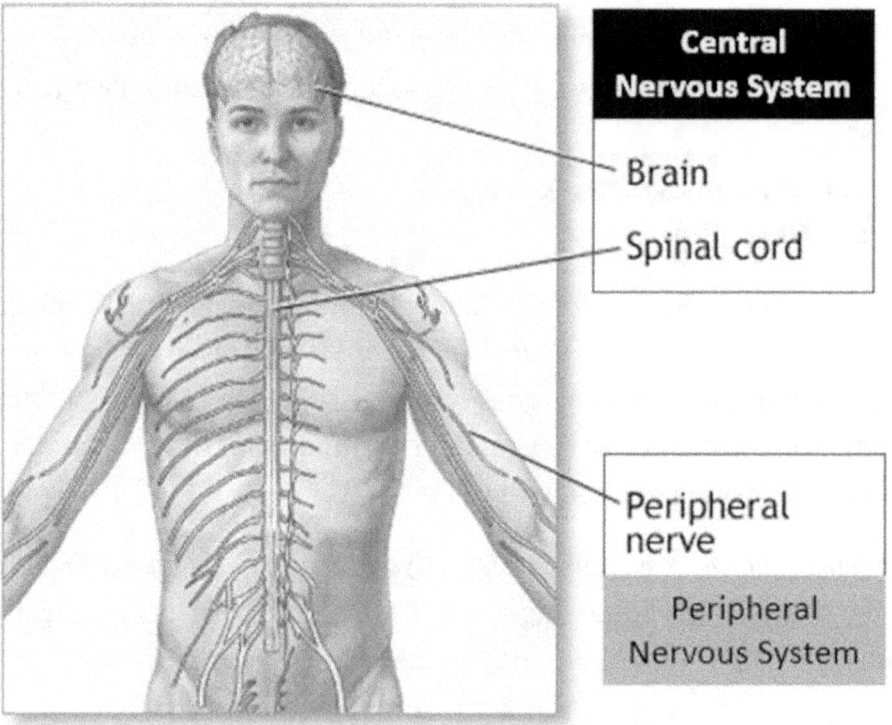

From the 'U.S. National Library of Medicine', Medline Plus.

If something goes wrong with the way the CNS handles the information it processes there will invariably be problems – consequential problems at that. The CNS may misinterpret information or get the processing wrong. Sometimes the CNS may believe, incorrectly, it has received information and attempt to process this 'phantom' information. This basically is what happens in the case of central pain syndrome. The CNS, *malfunctioning*, either misinterprets information it is receiving or starts dealing with 'phantom', non-existent information.

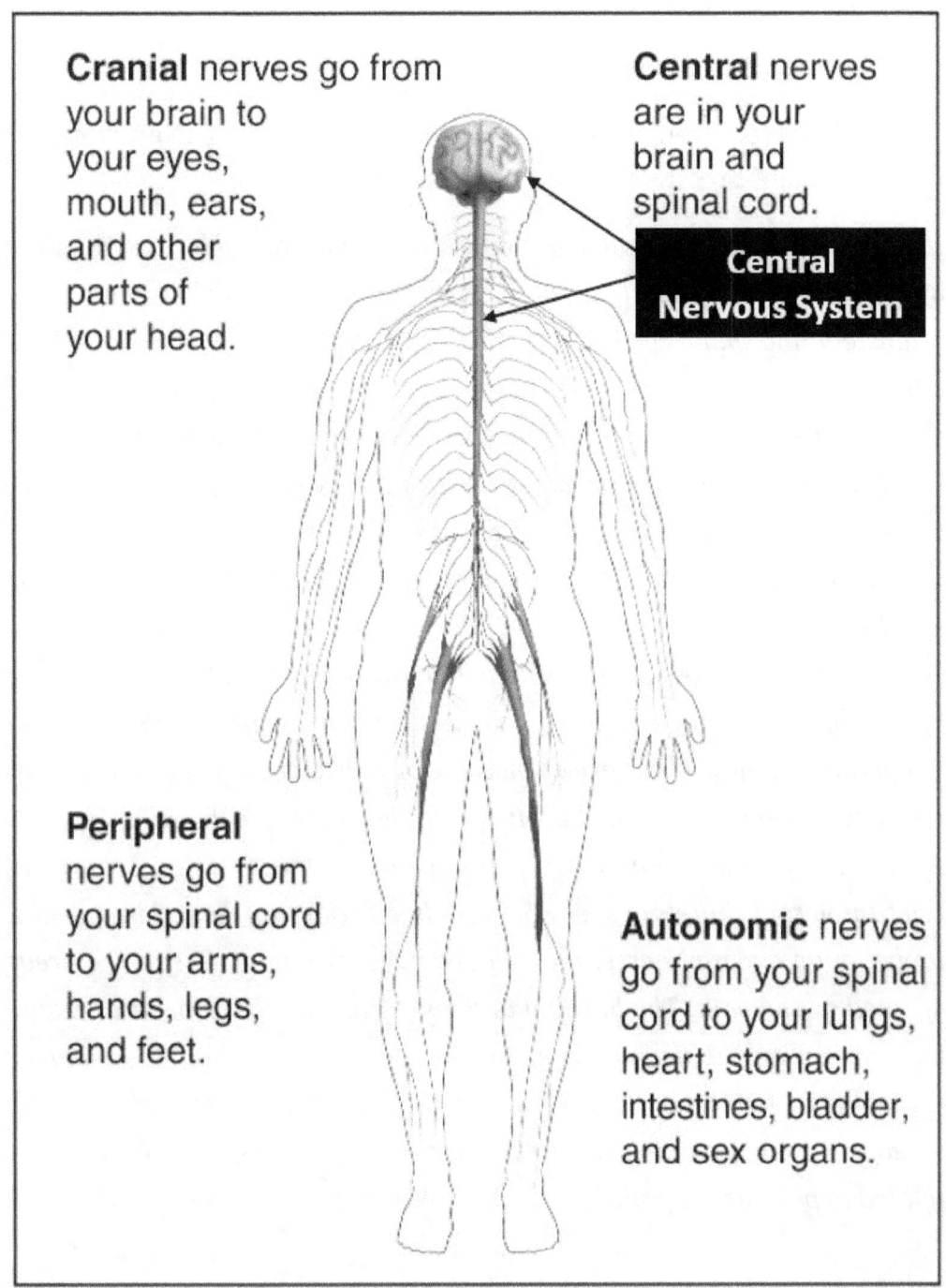

Cranial nerves go from your brain to your eyes, mouth, ears, and other parts of your head.

Central nerves are in your brain and spinal cord.

Central Nervous System

Peripheral nerves go from your spinal cord to your arms, hands, legs, and feet.

Autonomic nerves go from your spinal cord to your lungs, heart, stomach, intestines, bladder, and sex organs.

Base diagram from the U.S. government-funded 'National Center for Biotechnology Information' (NCBI).

There is more information on the Central Nervous System in *chapter 3, 'Possible Causes'*.

AN OFFICIAL DEFINITION OF
CENTRAL PAIN SYNDROME

The U.S. government-funded '**National Institute of Neurological Disorders and Stroke**' (NINDS) defines CPS as:

"Central pain syndrome is a neurological condition caused by damage to or dysfunction of the central nervous system (CNS), which includes the brain, brainstem, and spinal cord. This syndrome can be caused by stroke, multiple sclerosis, tumors, epilepsy, brain or spinal cord trauma, or Parkinson's disease. The character of the pain associated with this syndrome differs widely among individuals partly because of the variety of potential causes. Central pain syndrome may affect a large portion of the body or may be more restricted to specific areas, such as hands or feet. The extent of pain is usually related to the cause of the CNS injury or damage. Pain is typically constant, may be moderate to severe in intensity, and is often made worse by touch, movement, emotions, and temperature changes, usually cold temperatures. Individuals experience one or more types of pain sensations, the most prominent being burning. Mingled with the burning may be sensations of "pins and needles;" pressing, lacerating, or aching pain; and brief, intolerable bursts of sharp pain similar to the pain caused by a dental probe on an exposed nerve. Individuals may have numbness in the areas affected by the pain. The burning and loss of touch sensations are usually most severe on the distant parts of the body, such as the feet or hands. Central pain syndrome often begins shortly after the causative injury or damage, but may be delayed by months or even years, especially if it is related to post-stroke pain."

This is not a bad definition. It captures the essence of the syndrome and describes the most common symptoms. It also takes care to highlight, very early on, *both* the possible *variability* of the pain characteristics, and that the pain may be *local* <u>or</u> *widespread*.

It is worth reading this NINDS definition multiple times; slowly and thoughtfully. Then see how it fits in with your situation.

The first sentence is somewhat distracting in that it refers to *'neurological condition'* as well as *'damage to or dysfunction of the central nervous system'*. 'Neurological', by itself, however, is a reference to the nervous system.

So, that first sentence brings up the nervous system <u>twice</u>. And that is confirmation as to <u>how key</u> the central nervous system is to understanding this condition.

The bottom line, per this definition, being that this is a syndrome having to do with something that has *gone wrong in the brain, spinal cord or nervous system*. Coming to terms with that will help in understanding and coping with this exasperating and often debilitating condition.

The causes for CPS, listed in the second sentence, are, without doubt, the 'big ones' associated with this condition. But, there could be others. *Chapter 3* of this book is devoted to that topic, i.e., the possible causes.

WHY IS IT A SYNDROME?

'Syndrome' indicates there is a *combination* of symptoms associated with this condition.

If a condition can be identified with one specific symptom, then it is not a syndrome.

'Syndrome' highlights the spectrum of symptoms associated with CPS. If you have quite a few of the symptoms then there is a fairly good chance that you suffer from that syndrome, in this case CPS.

Since it is a syndrome, all CPS sufferers will not have the same set of symptoms. *The spectrum of symptoms being experienced could vary from one person to another.* However, each sufferer will typically have their own specific group of *predictable* symptoms – that can come and go, but persist over a long period of time.

'PMS' is a syndrome – Premenstrual *Syndrome.* As anybody familiar with PMS will agree, there are a lot of different symptoms, and they vary, greatly. [There are supposed to be over 200 different symptoms associated with PMS.]

'Chronic Fatigue' is also a syndrome as is 'Carpal Tunnel'. 'Down' (or also "Down's") is another well-known syndrome. "Parkinson's" is sometimes referred to as a syndrome.

'**Fibromyalgia**', another pain disorder increasingly seen as being related, in some way, with CPS, is also a syndrome. [*More later.*] Again, this is a condition defined in terms of the *'most common symptoms'*. And that is what characterizes syndromes. You have to deal with them in terms of the *'most common symptoms'*. If you suffer from CPS you will know what that is all about. It is never just one symptom on its own.

CPS SYMPTOMS

The symptoms of CPS are many, variable and *ever changeable.* There will typically be a complex *cocktail* of pain and other displeasing sensations – the ingredients different for each, and always liable to change.

Some of the pain and sensations experienced will be acute; others not as much. The symptoms could be *fickle*; likely not to be the same for any length of time. They could change during the course of a day, and from day to day.

One thing, however, is likely to be constant; if you suffer from CPS there usually will always be *'something distracting'* going on within you!

CPS can be life altering and can majorly impact one's quality and enjoyment of life. It can also lead to, or worsen psychological and emotional issues, such as anxiety and depression. It can sap strength and energy. *Fatigue*, both mental and physical, could become a major issue.

The cloud of words and phrases at the start of this chapter includes most of the main symptoms associated with Central Pain Syndrome. The next chapter, i.e., chapter 2, is devoted to the symptoms.

Some of the ingredients that could go into a CPS cocktail of discomfort include: pain of various sorts, burning, aching, numbness, tightness of muscles, itching, twitching, freezing, pins-and-needles, throbbing, cutting, ripping, tearing and tingling.

FIBROMYALGIA &
CENTRAL PAIN SYNDROME

That there is a connection between Fibromyalgia and CPS is hard to ignore. Many that eventually get diagnosed as suffering from CPS previously thought, or may have been told by doctors, that they had fibromyalgia. This is to be expected given they do share a large number of symptoms, especially chronic pain and tenderness involving muscles, bones, joints, tendons and ligaments – as well as fatigue, depression and anxiety.

The pain associated with fibromyalgia, as with CPS, can be widespread and sufferers invariably complain about *'aching all over'*. However, it *used to be the case* that doctors diagnosed fibromyalgia by checking for pain in 9 pairs (*18 points*) of 'tender spots'. [See diagram below.] If, upon pressure being applied, pain was felt in at least *11 of these points*, per the guidelines followed by doctors, a patient would be diagnosed as having fibromyalgia.

Of late there is <u>not</u> as much emphasis on this 9-pair checklist. It has been realized that the pain symptoms can be much more distributed – and that there is more to fibromyalgia, such as debilitating fatigue, sleep disorders and emotional distress, than just pain.

Fibromyalgia *used to be thought* of as a condition related to rheumatism (or arthritis). The name itself indicates that it has to do with pain in muscles and fibrous tissues (i.e., some of the body's connective tissues).

Fibromyalgia = *'Fibro'* (Latin for fibrous tissue) + *'myo'* (Greek for muscle) + *'algia'* (Latin for pain). *'Myalgia'*, by itself, is also a medical term and refers to pain in a specific muscle or a group of muscles.

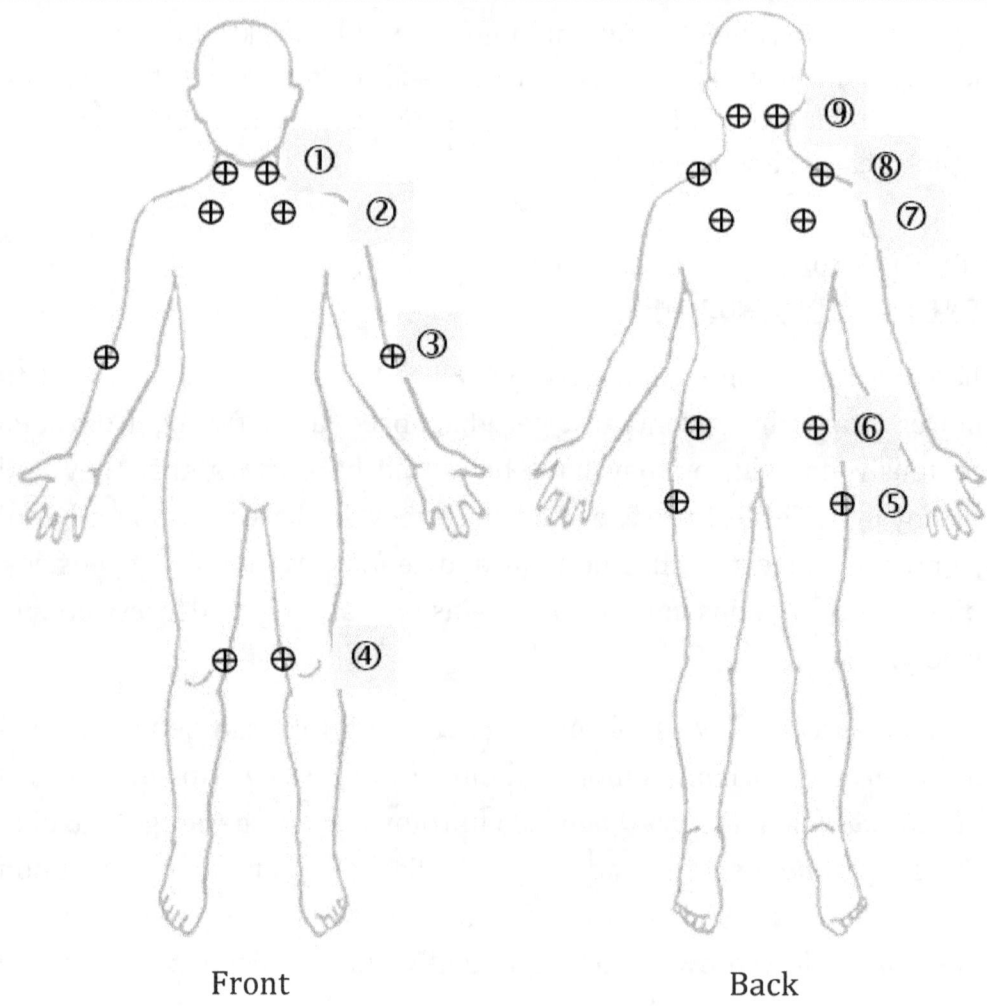

Front   Back

The 9 pairs (18 points) of tender points that *used to be* checked for fibromyalgia diagnosis.

Fibromyalgia, however, is *no longer* considered to be arthritis-related in that there is __no__ associated inflammation or damage to muscles, joints, tendons, or connective tissue! The latest thinking is that fibromyalgia, like CPS, is a central nervous system related disorder.

The 'Mayo Clinic' (in January 2017) states in the second sentence of its definition of fibromyalgia: '*... amplifies painful sensations by affecting the way your brain processes pain signals*'. Note the word '*processes*'.

The 'American College of Rheumatology' when talking about the causes of fibromyalgia states: *'... it is as though the "volume control" is turned up too high in the brain's pain processing centers'*. Again, note the *'processing'*.

The 'National Institute of Arthritis and Musculoskeletal and Skin Diseases' (a member of the U.S. 'National Institutes of Health') now says, in the section on 'causes': *'Many researchers are examining other causes, including problems with how the central nervous system (the brain and spinal cord) processes pain'.* This line of thinking is not all together new. It was initially suspected over 30 year ago. Within a few years of it first being identified as a specific condition there was talk that there might be an interconnection between fibromyalgia and other pain conditions.

On May 16, **2015**, the 'American Pain Society' issued a press release titled *'Fibromyalgia Has Central Nervous System Origins'*. Its opening sentence was: *'Fibromyalgia is the second most common rheumatic disorder behind osteoarthritis and, though still widely misunderstood, is now considered to be a lifelong central nervous system disorder, which is responsible for amplified pain that shoots through the body in those who suffer from it'.*

To cap it all, the 'National Fibromyalgia & Chronic Pain Association' (NfmCPA) has an article with the title: ***'Fibromyalgia: A Perfect Example of Centralized Pain'.***

While those that have been told that they have fibromyalgia may not know this, fibromyalgia is quite a controversial topic among medical professionals. Way back in 1987, the much respected *'Journal of the American Medical Association'* while coining the term *'fibromyalgia syndrome'* went onto add that it was a 'controversial condition'! One of the doctors who in 1990 had come up with the 18-point diagnostic guideline, stated in 2008 that he now believes that fibromyalgia is a body's response to *depression and stress* rather than a specific disease in its own right! Five years later he went onto add that its causes, in a sense, are controversial and that the symptoms could be due to a combination of psychological and physical issues.

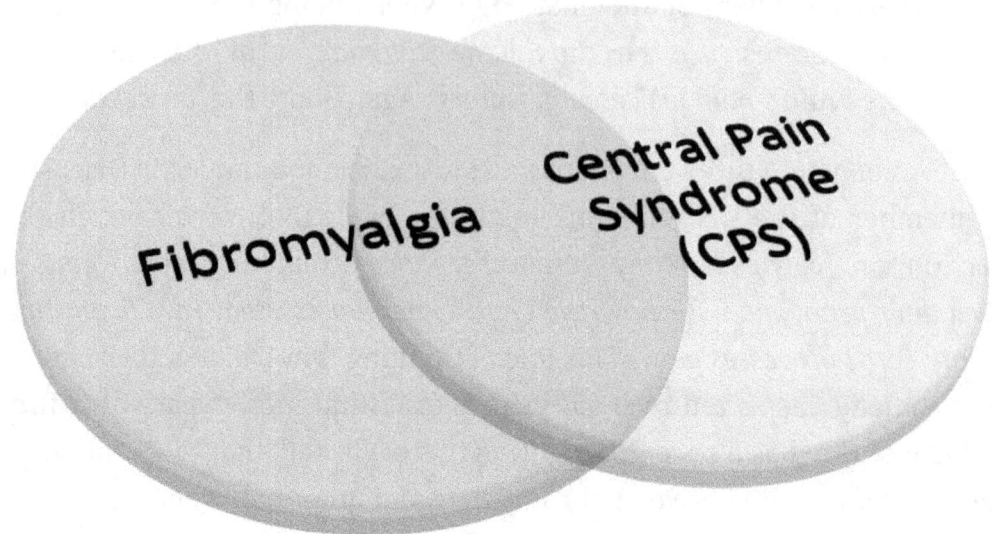

The *overlap* between fibromyalgia and Central Pain Syndrome (CPS).
The extent of this overlap has yet to be determined.
It could turn out to be quite high.

Thus, there is no longer much to be gained by debating whether one has central pain syndrome or fibromyalgia. The treatment regimens for both are essentially the same. The only real relevant distinction, particularly so in the U.S., might have to do with how one's health insurance covers one condition as opposed to the other. As such there could be instances when a doctor opts to document the condition as one or the other (typically fibromyalgia) to keep the insurance companies at bay.

So, there is this overlap between central pain syndrome and fibromyalgia. If you have fibromyalgia it might actually be CPS. Most of those with CPS more than likely could also be classed as having fibromyalgia. What has yet to be determined is the extent of the overlap. It could turn out to be that CPS and fibromyalgia are two sides of the same coin.

THE NUMBERS

It is estimated
(by the likes of the U.S. 'National Institutes of Health' (NIH))
that **5 million Americans**, 18 or older,
suffer from *fibromyalgia* –
well *over 75%* of these being <u>women</u>.

Some believe that the 5 million is too low
and the real number may be twice that.

There is, however, not as much reliable data,
at present, on the prevalence of Central Pain Syndrome.
Therefore, the best that is currently being said is that
over a ***few million people*** (in excess of 3 million),
worldwide, are believed to suffer from CPS.

The CPS number also could be much, much higher.

There is also no adequate data
on any gender bias.

In time, with a better understanding of
both CPS and fibromyalgia,
it *may be* determined that
CPS is more widespread than fibromyalgia.
Or, it may still be the case that
fibromyalgia, or at least the diagnosis of it,
is more widespread.

CENTRAL PAIN SYNDROME & CHRONIC PAIN (SYNDROME)

Chronic pain refers to persistent, long-term pain lasting 6 months or longer. Some set the threshold at 3 months. In either case, pain that lasts less than that is called 'acute' or 'subacute'. CPS, which is invariably a lifelong condition, obviously qualifies as 'chronic pain' – irrespective of whether the threshold is 3 or 6 months.

Chronic pain is further subdivided into two categories:

1. Pain caused by inflamed or damaged tissue, and

2. Pain caused by damage or malfunction of the *nervous system*.

By now you will know that the second category relates to CPS. So, that is a second intersection between chronic pain and CPS.

The 'syndrome' associated with chronic pain, as with CPS, has to do with the multiple, varied symptoms. WebMD, when describing chronic pain, has this to say in its very first paragraph: *'Pain signals are somehow triggered by the nervous system and continue to fire for months or even years. (It is also possible that certain brain chemicals that suppress pain do not work properly.)'* Notice the similarity to the wording used when talking about CPS.

As with fibromyalgia, in the end, from a practical, treatment-oriented perspective, it does not really matter whether you are diagnosed as having chronic pain syndrome or central pain syndrome – provided that your pain is <u>NOT</u> caused by inflamed or damaged tissues or joints. As long as it is indeed the case, what really matters is the recognition that your pain is due to a CNS disorder. There is really not much difference in how the two syndromes are treated – with doctors in general, trying in both cases, to treat some of the most bothersome symptoms.

CENTRAL SENSITIZATION SYNDROME

'*Central sensitization*' is a new term that is being used to describe how and why the nervous system *succumbs* to '*chronic pain*' – whether it be CPS or something else.

The basis of '*central sensitization*' is that <u>*persistent pain, on its own*</u>, over time ends up <u>*conditioning*</u> the central nervous system to be <u>*more sensitive to pain*</u>.

Got that? **Self-perpetuating pain**. Persistent pain leading to more pain. The CNS reacting over time to be *more sensitive to ALL pain* – such that it creates **more pain** with **less instigation**.

Those with CPS will be able to relate to this (once they work out what is really happening inside their body). This is why things that shouldn't normally be painful, like a light touch or the feeling of clothing, now end up causing noticeable pain.

Central sensitization contends that persistent pain results in the CNS getting '*wound up*' – elevating it to a state where it is more sensitive, reactive and 'on edge'. This is what used to get described as the '*volume being turned up*' when it came to pain.

Central sensitization is becoming the umbrella under which much of the current (and possibly future) research into chronic pain is being conducted. So, add '*central sensitization (syndrome)*' to your vocabulary and 'watch list'. Any advances they make in better understanding and treating central sensitization will be applicable to CPS. The next time you see your pain doctor bring up central sensitization. Going forward it is best if CPS was looked at and treated within the context of both chronic pain and central sensitization syndrome.

TAKEAWAYS:
CHAPTER 1 – AN OVERVIEW

- ᛭ Central Pain Syndrome (CPS) is caused by *damage to* or *dysfunction of* the **central** nervous system (CNS) – i.e., the brain and the spinal cord.

- ᛭ CPS is the eventual result of some kind of prior violation to one's brain and/or spinal cord, e.g., brain or spinal injury.

- ᛭ The pain/burning symptoms of CPS are not caused by any harmful injury, impact or damage to the body. Instead it is pain that originates in the brain, due to a disruption to how the brain processes pain in general.

- ᛭ That CPS is a 'syndrome' just indicates that there is a combination of symptoms associated with it. PMS, fibromyalgia, chronic fatigue and 'Down' are also all syndromes.

- ᛭ The symptoms of CPS are many, variable and ever changing. It is a complex *cocktail* of pain and unpleasant sensations – with ingredients specific to each sufferer and, furthermore, liable to frequent and arbitrary changes.

- ᛭ The symptoms of CPS are fickle, but more often than not, are likely to be unrelenting.

- ᛭ There is an undeniable connection between CPS and fibromyalgia. Given that the treatment for both are essentially identical, it does not, in practice, make much difference as to whether you are told you have one or the other – insurance coverage, possibly, the only concern.

- ᛭ CPS, invariably a lifelong condition, falls under the nervous system-related category of *Chronic Pain Syndrome*.

> You have to always think of CPS in terms of *central nervous system*, rather than in terms of the various pains and sensations.

2.
THE SYMPTOMS

Pain in some form, relentless and seemingly unending, is the most common, telltale indication. In some instances, there may, however, be short periods of temporary relief – with the pain symptoms going away for a period of time, albeit to always *come back*.

The intensity of the pain can fluctuate between tolerable to intolerable. On the 0-to-10 pain scale used by doctors, the pain much of the time will be at or above 4, and will rarely (if ever) go down below 2. Periods of *excruciating pain*, usually of short duration, is relatively common. The intensity of the pain can be such that some have described it as being '*shocking*' – the **worst** they have ever experienced, even more intense than anything experienced in a dentist's chair.

When not at its highest *agonizing* intensity the pain may come across as an *aching*, *crushing* or *pressing* sensation.

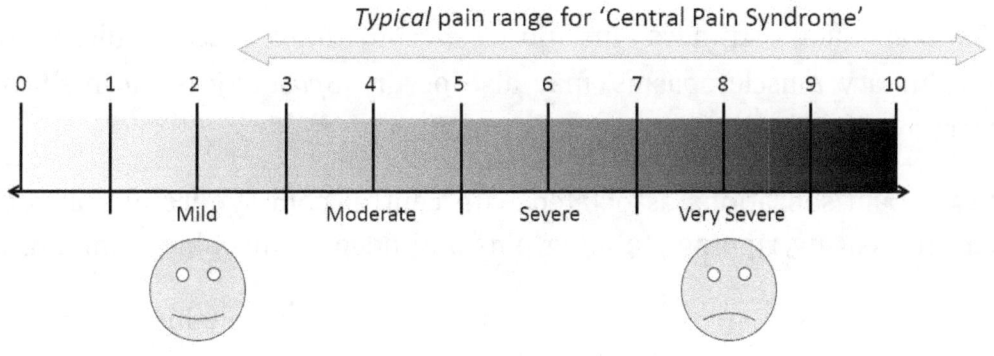

The pain can be *local* or *widespread*. It may be restricted to certain parts of the body, e.g., just the limbs, or occur in various, different parts of the body – *all at once*. It may hurt more in some areas than others. Hence, why it is a 'syndrome'. If brought about as a result of a <u>stroke</u> the symptoms may, however, always be restricted to just one side of the body.

CPS is a condition that defies specifics or generalization. The one exception being that the symptoms will be very specific to each sufferer.

Burning sensations are another widespread characteristic. The feeling of <u>*persistent*</u> burning is often considered to be the *most telling* clue to CPS. To confound matters sensations of *freezing* may be interspersed with those of burning! Severe, inexplicable itching is yet another possibility. [The medical term for this itching is *pruritus*.] *Tingling* and *prickling* are also not uncommon.

Touching or even the feel of clothes (or bedding) can make the pain/burning/freezing/itching sensations feel worse. Sometimes this skin-level sensitivity could be so acute that even a moderate amount of *air movement* from a fan or the wind can be aggravating.

Changes in *temperature*, especially a drop-in temperature, can worsen all the symptoms, especially that of pain.

Numbness, particularly of the face, feet and hands, is another frequent telltale occurrence. Weakness in a limb, maybe related to numbness, is also possibility. Some sufferers complain that the numbness is such that it hurts!

Tightness and stiffness in muscles, sometimes accompanied by involuntary muscle spasms, may also occur. [*Spasticity* is the medical term for these muscle-related abnormalities.]

Other pain sensations associated with central pain syndrome include: cutting, tearing, ripping, stabbing, pins-and-needles, throbbing, tingling …

CPS caused by a <u>stroke</u> could also result in uncontrollable, unnatural twitching, jerkiness and twisting of limbs and face.

Variability, different *cocktails of symptoms*, and *shades-of-grey* are all hallmarks of CPS. Each sufferer will have their own grab bag of symptoms – at any given time. The symptoms and the combinations in which they occur can change over time – even during the course of a day.

With CPS you feel that you never get a break. There always appears to be something unpleasant going on, somewhere.

In females, hormones can dramatically influence the symptoms. In those of menstruating age, the symptoms may worsen around the time of ovulation. This should not be overlooked.

Stress or physical exertion can aggravate the symptoms. Certain movements or any type of travel may also be problematic. Rest often helps reduce the severity of the symptoms, as do, on occasion, pleasurable distractions, hobbies and pastimes. But, the motivation to pursue hobbies and pastimes may become hard to muster. Depression could make everything worse.

OCCURRENCE

Central pain syndrome is caused by some sort of *violation* to the *central nervous system*, i.e., to the brain or the spinal cord. [The next chapter deals with all the possible causes.]

As to when the symptoms of CPS may start to appear following a violation can *vary widely*. It could be within a *few hours* or it might be after a *few years*! There is no set time period.

Delayed onset can be confounding, especially if there was an expectation that a violation to the central nervous system was in the process of being healed (e.g., spinal surgery to help a spinal disc injury). Hence it may take some effort to determine what may have caused the onset of CPS.

The degree of severity of the original violation does not appear to influence the severity of the CPS symptoms. All that appears to matter is that there was some form of trauma to the central nervous system at *some point in the past*. Thus, it is possible that even what was a relatively minor violation may cause excruciating CPS symptoms. There is no fairness, whatsoever, when it comes to CPS.

There could be a gradual but incessant build-up of symptoms or it could all begin with a bang.

Until they are diagnosed as being CPS-related the symptoms of CPS will initially defy explanation. The symptoms, e.g., the pain, burning, itching or numbness, would appear to be without cause – with nothing definite that the patient or a doctor can identify as triggering the symptoms. As such the term '*spontaneous*' will often be seen in medical literature in reference to the symptoms of CPS.

The cocktail of symptoms can – and in many instances, will – change; during the course of the day, from day-to-day, and over time. The treatment being undertaken could be a factor. Some symptoms might go away to be replaced by others. It could become a cat-and-mouse game.

In general, once you start suffering from CPS it is unlikely to go away. It is, alas, considered to be a lifelong condition with no magical, silver-bullet cure. But, there can be periods of remission – however, slight.

OTHER COMPLICATIONS

Central pain syndrome, more often than not, is a lifestyle changing disorder.

It is quite common that the toll of dealing with CPS will cause psychological distress. Thus, CPS can cause, or worsen, anxiety and depression.

Trying to cope with the never-ending, ever changing pains, aches and sensations of CPS can be demanding, taxing and exhausting. It will make some distracted, preoccupied and withdrawn. There could be frequent mood swings and feelings of irrational, intense anger.

Increased fatigue, or even chronic fatigue, is another possibility. CPS sufferers will often talk about how tired they feel – all the time.

In some instances, CPS, with or without the added psychological complications, could be crippling.

CPS sufferers, over time, are likely to become oversensitive, or even hypersensitive, to pain. Pain that they previously would have been able to tolerate quite well would now become unbearable. Those that may have previously claimed *'I have a high tolerance to pain'* will cease to say so – or feel so. Things that may not be painful (or distressing) to others, such as being touched on the arm or shoulder, can be painful to those suffering from CPS.

This hypersensitivity is a major feature of CPS. But, it is something that is easy to overlook or underestimate – particularly since increased pain makes one distracted and preoccupied. When dealing with acute pain one is not inclined to think about whether some of the pain is due to the hypersensitivity of CPS. That is an issue. The pain becomes all consuming – which in turn could make the hypersensitivity worse! This is the so called '**central sensitization**' described at the end of chapter 1.

Pain becomes a vicious-cycle – fed by hypersensitivity. Refer to chapter 4, *'Pain & The Brain'*.

WITH CPS PAIN BECOMES A DOMINANT FACTOR OF LIFE.

Pain clouds outlook, judgement and decisions. Everything gets viewed through a prism of pain. All plans and decisions are filtered through a lens of pain – negativity, in terms of an unwillingness to do 'things', becoming a consistent theme.

CPS can definitely degrade a person's quality of life – quite severely. Some may find that it interferes with their ability to perform routine, daily tasks – and as such get on with normal life. And, of course, the impediments of CPS will not be restricted just to those suffering from it. CPS will affect family and friends of those affected – particularly those living with a sufferer. CPS will negatively impact entire households. CPS will leave a long legacy of pain – much of it psychological. *CPS sucks.*

TAKEAWAYS:
CHAPTER 2 – THE SYMPTOMS

- ✍ Pain in some form -- local or widespread -- unyielding, unforgiving and seemingly never ending, is a hallmark of Central Pain Syndrome.

- ✍ Long lasting *burning sensations* are often a telltale symptom.

- ✍ Numbness, as well as muscle stiffness is common.

- ✍ The intensity of the pain and other unpleasant sensations will fluctuate, often and unpredictably – with no rhyme or reason other than, apparently, to exasperate.

- ✍ Changes in temperature can aggravate symptoms.

- ✍ Being lightly touched, the feel of clothing/bedding or even a gentle breeze may become intolerable.

- ✍ Those that suffer from CPS, over time, can become *oversensitive*, or even *hypersensitive*, to pain. This is the so called '*sensitization*' of the pain system – the amplification of the brain's response to **ALL** pain signals, **NOT** *just the pain associated with CPS*. Central Sensitization.

- ✍ As to when CPS may occur following a violation to the central nervous system can vary widely; it could be hours, it could be years. Also, worth noting that all violations do not result in CPS.

- ✍ CPS, invariably a lifelong condition, can, and most likely will, be lifestyle changing – 'debilitating', an oft used term when it comes to CPS.

- ✍ Coping with CPS, which can be demanding, taxing and exhausting, can cause psychological distress – and make one distracted, preoccupied, withdrawn and quick to anger.

- ✍ CPS can become the dominant factor of a sufferer's life.

3.
POSSIBLE CAUSES

For you to have Central Pain Syndrome there *had to have been* some type of prior violation to the central nervous system. Of that there is no doubt, debate or disagreement.

Possible violations to the central nervous system (i.e., brain/brainstem and spinal cord) that could *eventually* result in CPS *include*:

❖ A **stroke**.

❖ Multiple sclerosis (**MS**).

❖ **Head injuries**, including some forms of concussion.

❖ **Spinal cord injury**, which includes damage to *vertebrae*, *disks* or ligaments of the *spinal column*.

❖ **Tumors**: brain tumors, spinal tumors and those close to any part of the central nervous system – including *cancerous* growths.

❖ **Epilepsy**.

❖ Neurosurgical procedures or **surgeries** involving the spine or brain.

❖ **Aneurysms**: brain aneurysms in particular, but also aneurysms affecting the central nervous system.

❖ **Parkinson's disease**.

❖ **Infections** of the central nervous system, which could be *viral, bacterial, fungal,* etc., and includes conditions such as: **meningitis** (in various forms), tuberculosis (TB), late stage **Lyme disease**, malaria, encephalitis (in various forms), rabies, **shingles**, brain abscesses, leprosy and Guillain–Barré syndrome (GBS). The list of central nervous system-related infections is long and involves quite a few obscure conditions – e.g., different types of encephalitis. Those mentioned above are just some of the better known. A longer list, though probably still not fully complete, can be found at Wikipedia under *'list of infections of the central nervous system'*. This list will be a good list to start with if you suspect that you may have had an infection that may have led to CPS.

Central Pain Syndrome *is not* a condition that *ever* develops on its own. It is always considered to be a *secondary event*. An unwelcome, unpleasant **aftereffect** or **side effect** of an earlier condition.

The medical term for the nature of CPS is *sequela* – a condition that is a consequence of a prior disease or injury. It is from the Latin for 'sequel'.

It is indeed possible that multiple causes are responsible for one's CPS, for example, a prior spinal cord injury followed by a stroke, or late stage Lyme and a head injury. If you have CPS (or was in the process of getting CPS), your pain system would already be hypersensitive – reacting, adversely, to any new cause of pain or distress. So, the above causes could be *cumulative* – though in practice that is unlikely to be that relevant in trying to deal with CPS. CPS due to just one cause is likely to be as unpleasant and hard to deal with as CPS due to multiple causes!

STROKE RELATED

It is believed that **8 – 12%** of those that suffer a stroke end up having CPS.

In some circles this condition is known as *Central Stroke Pain* or *Central Poststroke Pain* (CPSP). It also used to be known as *Dejerine-Roussy Syndrome* or *Thalamic Pain Syndrome.*

Joseph Jules Dejerine and Gustave Roussy were French neurologists who identified this condition, relative to strokes, in 1906. Central pain itself, however, had been identified by a German neurologist, Ludwig Edinger, in **1891**. 'Thalamic', a term used by Dejerine and Roussy in the title of their 1906 paper, refers to an area inside of the brain known as the **'Thalamus'**. See picture below. *The thalamus is like the brain's router.* It is responsible for processing sensory information and routing that information to other parts of the brain. So, you can see why CPS, as a central nervous system disorder, would be associated with the thalamus.

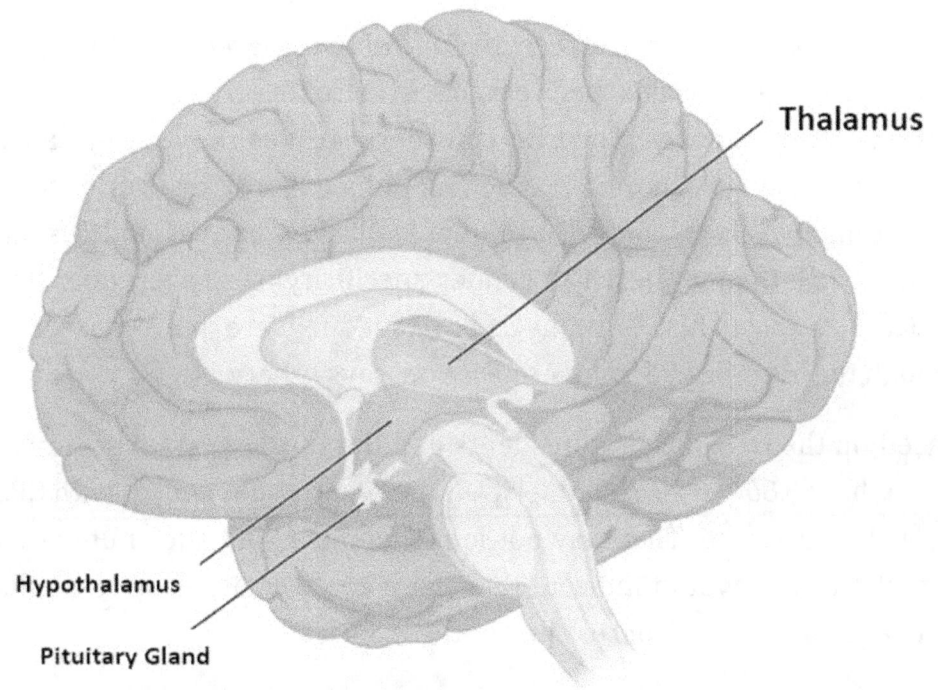

A *cutaway* diagram of the brain showing the thalamus
which is in the 'middle' of the brain, surrounded
by the right and left brain hemispheres.

From 'OpenStax' (at 'Rice University')
via cnx.org.

CPS-related symptoms typically show up a few weeks after a stroke. The most common symptoms tend to be pain, numbness and an assortment of 'weird' sensations. Hypersensitivity, particularly to temperature change and cold temperatures, is widespread.

Strokes are more common than most people realize. Though there are no accurate numbers, it is believed that first-time incidence of strokes *per year*, *worldwide*, are in the region of 17 million. That means somebody, somewhere, is having a stroke, for the first time, *every two seconds*!

If 8 – 12% of these that suffered a first-time stroke end up with CPS, that would mean *1.4 to 2 million folks a year*, worldwide, join the ranks of CPS sufferers due to stroke.

In the U.S., per *'Centers for Disease Control and Prevention'* (CDC), more than 795,000 Americans, per year, have a stroke – 610,000 of these are first (or 'new') strokes. The CDC considers strokes the leading cause of long-term disability in the U.S. The risk of having a stroke varies by race and ethnicity; blacks, American Indians, Alaskan natives and Hispanics more at risk than whites. The gender-specificity of strokes, however, is apparently inconclusive. Many claim that men are more susceptible, though the 'American Stroke Association' says otherwise.

Based on the 610,000 first incidents and the 8 – 12% statistic, it would mean that *48,800* to *73,200* Americans, per year, could end up with CPS as a result of a stroke. That may not look like much, but such numbers are cumulative and would indicate that there could easily be over a million stroke-induced CPS sufferers just in the U.S.

The 'Mayo Clinic' Website, of course, covers 'stroke'. The CPS-related symptoms are discussed in the section on 'Complications' under the subheading 'Pain'. This section (at least in January 2017) concludes with this sentence: *"But because the pain is caused by a problem in your brain, rather than a physical injury, there are few treatments"*. While the claim about 'few treatments' maybe too overly dire, the thrust of this sentence is worth keeping in mind.

That sentence sets out to stress that CPS is due to a problem in *your brain* – as opposed to physical injury or inflammation at the *apparent site* of the pain.

One needs to always come back to this '*in your brain*' notion when trying to cope with the distress of CPS. It is also important when trying to evaluate treatment options. The pain, burning or twitching may be in your arm, foot or neck, but the real problem is not in your arm, foot or neck. It is something awry within the central nervous system that is causing the pain. And as such, when it comes to CPS, it is always the central nervous system (CNS) that has to be dealt with and appeased.

MULTIPLE SCLEROSIS (MS)

Multiple sclerosis, often leading to debilitation, is a disease of the central nervous system. Thus, it should not be surprising that those that have MS could also end up with CPS symptoms – given that CPS arises from damage to or dysfunction of the CNS.

It is believed that **20%** of those with MS experience symptoms of CPS.

With MS, the insulation that protects nerve cells get attacked – and hence damaged – by the body's immune system. It is, as such, *believed* to be an autoimmune disease (where the body's immune system mistakenly starts to attack healthy cells) though there is still some debate as to this -- or whether it is the only cause.

This damage to the insulation (known as 'myelin') disrupts information flow to/from the CNS, as well as within the CNS. Progressive disintegration of the insulation layer (or 'sheath' as it is often called) can lead to permanent nerve damage. Depending on the nerves involved, the extent of the nerve damage will determine the level of debilitation.

'Sclerosis' is a Greek word meaning 'hard'. The damage to the insulation causes parts of the nerve to harden. Hence, the name. It is also sometimes referred to as 'Focal Sclerosis'. The crippling nature of MS was being documented as long ago as the 1830s; it being recognized as a specific condition in the 1860s.

It is not unusual for those that start getting symptoms of CPS, as a result of a previous spinal cord or brain injury, to believe that they may have MS. There are, however, certain tests that can be used, conclusively, to diagnose MS. These include: blood tests for particular types of white blood cells, lumber punctures, medical imaging to detect hardening of nerves, and electrical measurements of the nervous system. It is worth noting that *there aren't as specific tests* for accurately diagnosing CPS – though medical imaging, such as MRIs, can be used to locate tumors or damage in and around the CNS. In most instances the diagnosis of CPS is achieved through the *elimination* of other possibilities, followed by then associating it to a *known compromise* of the central nervous system.

It is estimated that there are about 2.5 million people, worldwide, with MS – around 400,000 of these in the U.S. About 200 new cases, per week, are diagnosed in the U.S. There are twice as many women with MS than men. Though not considered to be a condition that is inherited, there seems to be a genetic factor involved – with people with North European ancestry most at risk.

Though the reason has yet to be determined, MS appears to have a very distinct geographic bias! It is definitely more prevalent the further one gets from the equator, and more so in the Northern Hemisphere than in the Southern. Northern states in the U.S. (above the 37th parallel, which starts in the east around the Virginia, North Carolina boundary) have *twice* as many cases of MS than those in the south. Canada has even more!

In Europe, the highest incidents of MS are in: Denmark, Sweden, Hungary, Norway, Czech Republic, U.K. and Germany. Yes, colder climes are inescapably a factor. It is even claimed that relocating to a lower risk area, prior to puberty, can reduce one's risks.

THE BRAIN & BRAIN STEM

The brain (including the brain stem) working in conjunction with the nervous system is the body's command and control center. It is worth referring to the full body diagram in chapter 1 (i.e., the 2nd figure in that chapter), if you are not that familiar with how the nervous system spreads out across your body – starting from the brain.

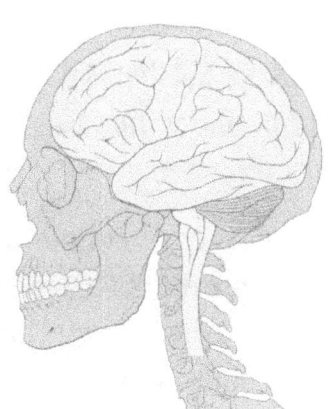

Though the skin and liver are larger and heavier, the brain (including the stem), undoubtedly, is THE body's most vital organ. It is the brain/brain stem, in the end, that controls and regulates breathing, heart rate, blood pressure, body temperature, digestion, sexual arousal and waste disposal. Without the brain we will not be able to see, hear, smell, taste or maintain our balance. Touch, and with that feel, not to mention thinking and learning, are also all brain related. *As is pain.* Suffice to say that any malfunctioning of the brain can have major consequences to one's life.

The cruciality of the brain when it comes to the body's wellbeing is such that brain death is widely used, around the world, as a legal definition of death. In the U.S., per the 1981 '*Uniform Determination of Death Act*', brain death is one of just two ways of determining death – the other being '*irreversible cessation of circulatory and respiratory functions*'. [This is somewhat of a circular definition in that brain death will result in the cessation of normal, unaided breathing, i.e., a brain-dead person can only breath when connected to a breathing machine.]

The brain plays a crucial role when it comes to CPS. That is inescapable. *If the brain would cooperate one could overcome CPS.* But, that is easier said than done, and in most instances unlikely to ever happen.

In terms of understanding CPS or dealing with CPS, it is not necessary to know how the brain functions, the different parts of the brain, or the responsibilities of each part. It is useful, however, to have a good mental image of the entire central nervous system – and the appreciation that all of the body's sensory information handling and processing is done within the CNS. So, that is what we will concentrate on. If you want to know more about the brain, there is no shortage of material on the Web and in book form.

The next chapter does deal with the *vital 'brain-pain' connection* so key in the context of CPS, while the '*Glossary*' towards the end of this book does include brief descriptions of the major parts of the brain, e.g., cerebrum, cerebellum and hypothalamus.

The thick bones of the skull provide the brain with its primary protection from external forces such as blows to the head or hitting the head against a hard surface. In addition, the brain is surrounded by three layers of membrane – which provide a relatively thin, but durable sheathing. These membranes are known as the *meninges*. **Meningitis**, a possible trigger for CPS, is an infection of the meninges. Any damage to the meninges, including hemorrhages, could result, down the road, in CPS.

The brain, furthermore, for added protection is surrounded by, and suspended in, a fluid. This fluid is known as the *cerebrospinal fluid*. This fluid and the meninges together form an isolating barrier between the brain and the rest of the body, including the blood stream. Everything that goes in and out of the brain is thus filtered through this combined barrier. Despite these protective layers, the brain, as we know, is susceptible to injury, infections, tumors and disease. Any of these, as listed at the start of this chapter, can result in CPS.

Brain Stem

The brain stem, located towards the rear of the brain, is what connects the rest of the brain with the spinal cord. Hence, its relevance to CPS. The central nervous system, at the very core of CPS, is defined as consisting of the brain and the spinal cord. The brain stem is the part that brings them together; what connects the spinal cord to the brain.

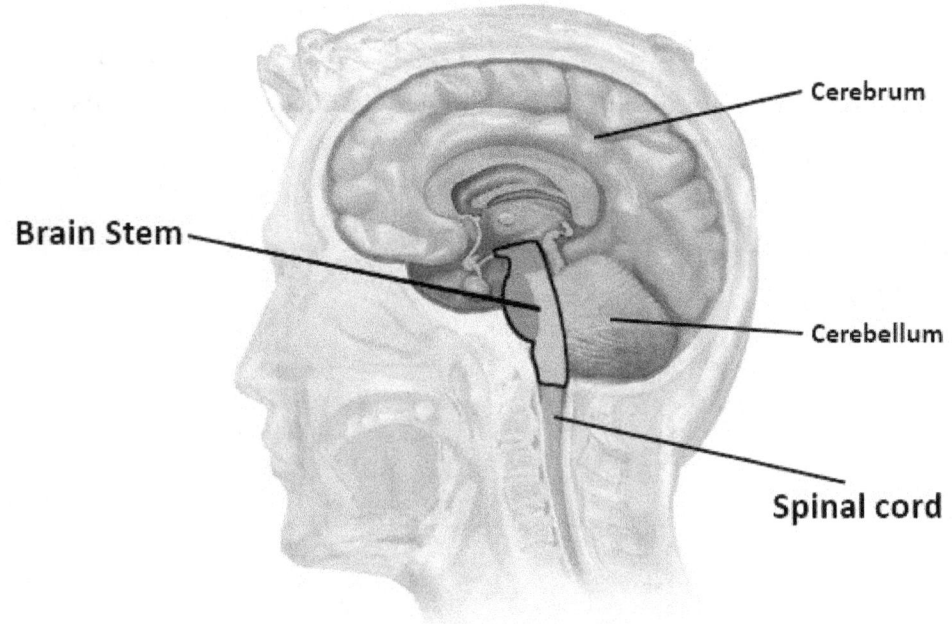

Another *cutaway* diagram. The brain stem, which consists of three parts, is outlined in black.

The brain stem is a cylindrical structure, slightly longer than 3", made up of nervous tissue. **Nervous tissue** (a.k.a. nerve tissue) is the main component of the nervous system – the combination of the central nervous system (CNS) and the peripheral nervous system.

Though its composition is not as complex as other parts of the brain, the brain stem is absolutely vital to survival.

The brain stem (a.k.a. 'brainstem') is part of the brain. However, it is sometimes mentioned separately of the brain – particularly in the context of the central nervous system.

Given that it is the connection between the spinal cord and the brain, all the nerves related to the body's sensory and motor (i.e., motion) functions pass through the brain stem. In addition, ten of the twelve pairs of nerves that originate in the brain, rather than in the spinal cord, and control sensory and motor functions to do with the face and neck, start off from the brain stem.

The brain stem plays a key role in managing: breathing, heart rate, blood pressure, body temperature, state of consciousness, sleep patterns, reflex coordination, and the feelings of hunger and thirst. *It is also responsible for regulating the central nervous system.* Hence, why the brain stem so often comes up in medical discussions related to CPS.

THE SPINAL CORD

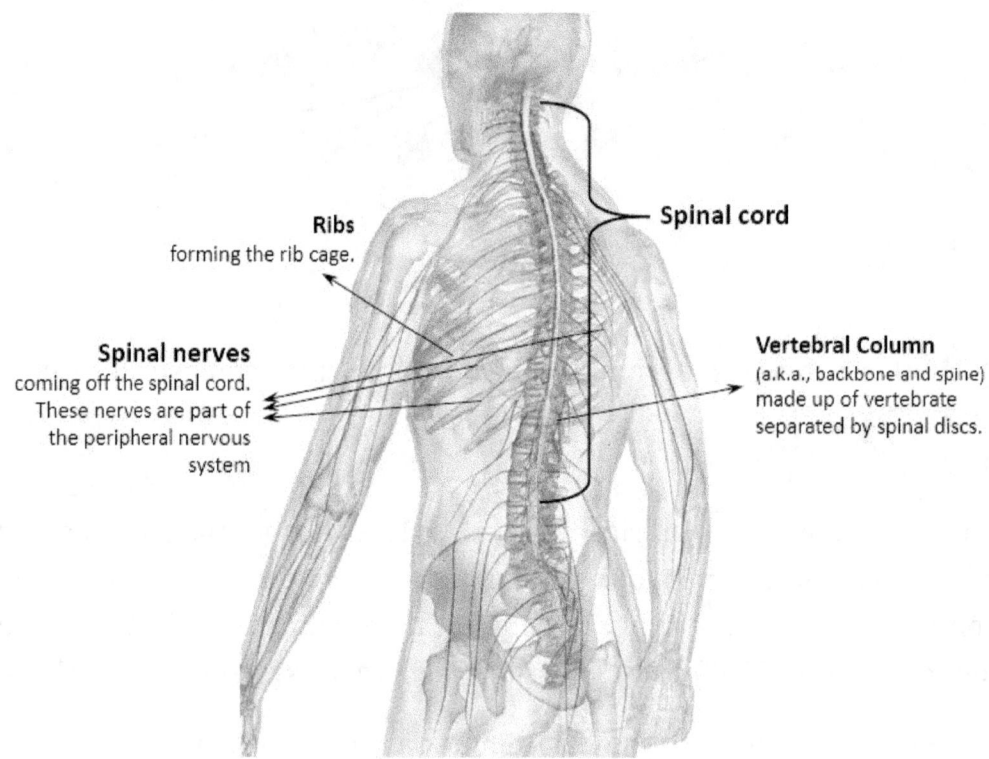

Ribs
forming the rib cage.

Spinal cord

Spinal nerves
coming off the spinal cord.
These nerves are part of
the peripheral nervous
system

Vertebral Column
(a.k.a., backbone and spine)
made up of vertebrate
separated by spinal discs.

The spinal cord is a thin (¼" to ½" wide) cylindrical bundle of nervous tissue, and support/protective cells – such as the cells that provide insulation and help in repairing damaged nerves.

The spinal cord runs from the bottom of your skull to your lumbar region, i.e., the area between your last rib and the pelvis. It does not extend all the way to the end of your spine (i.e., backbone or vertebral column). As such the spinal cord is not that long. The average length of the spinal column in men is around 18", while it is about one-inch shorter for women. [If that sounds too short, measure the distance. You will be surprised.]

The spinal cord is the primary path for information flow between the brain and the peripheral nervous system. It is, as such, the most important interface between your brain and your body.

The spinal cord, on its own, also controls various bodily reflexes and maintains certain repetitive rhythms such as that involved in walking.

The same type of three-layer membrane, as well as the same fluid, that form a protective barrier around the brain also protect the spinal cord. Together they form the inner layer of protection for the spinal cord. The *vertebral column* (i.e., spinal column or backbone), however, is the main protective mechanism for the spinal cord. *The vertebral column encases the delicate spinal column within its hard, bony structure.*

The vertebral column is made up primarily of vertebrae and spinal discs. There is an oval-shaped opening in the vertebra to accommodate and envelope the spinal cord. These oval-shaped openings form a tunnel within the spinal column, albeit with fairly large gaps on the side. The spinal cord resides inside this encasing tunnel. *The gaps (or openings) on the side enable the spinal nerves to exit the confines of the spinal column.*

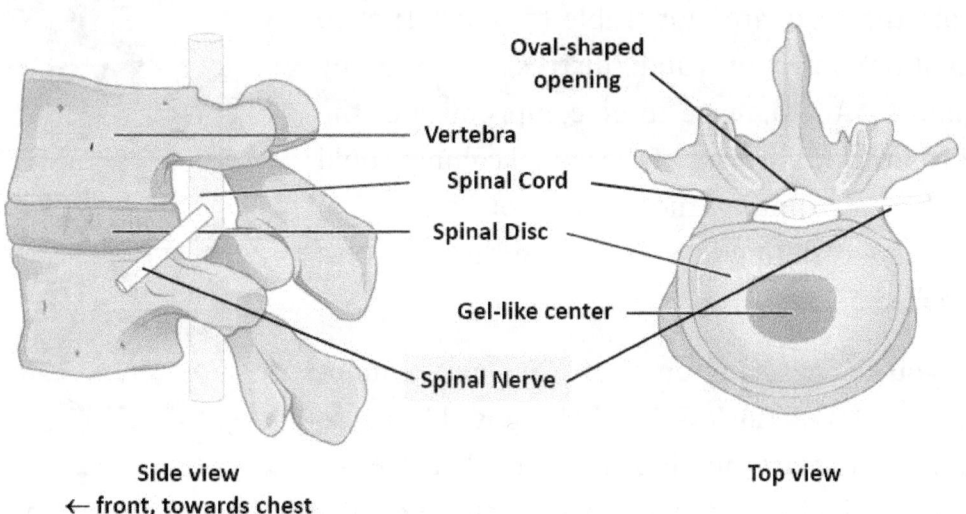

Side view
← front, towards chest

Top view

Notice from the diagram above that the spinal discs do not surround the spinal cord or the spinal nerves. Spinal discs sit in front of the spinal cord, in between the vertebrae. They act as cushioning, shock-absorbers. But, they are close enough to both the spinal cord and the spinal nerves to invade their space if a disc gets damaged – 'crushed', displaced or herniated (i.e., when the gel-like substance in the middle of the disc escapes through a tear in the disc). This is the cause of back trouble due to a pinched nerve or a crushed disk.

The spinal cord reaches all the way down to the L1 and L2 lumbar vertebrae on your spinal column. (Please refer to diagram.)

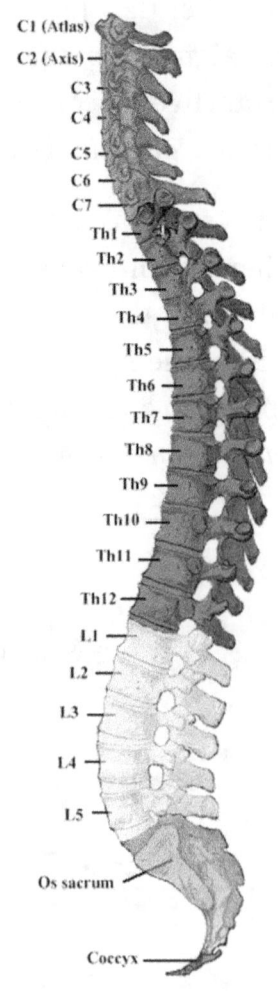

Whichever way you want to look at it, Central Pain Syndrome, per what is known at present, is considered to be, totally, a central nervous system-related condition. PERIOD. The central nervous system is made up of just *two parts* – and one of them is the spinal cord. Despite the protection afforded by the spinal column, the spinal cord, and the spinal nerves branching out from the cord, are vulnerable to injury (not to mention infection and distress caused by tumors). Any damage to or compromise of the vertebrae or the discs of the spinal column could end up disrupting the spinal cord or spinal nerves – resulting in pressure on the cord or a pinched nerve.

If you have symptoms of CPS but cannot immediately associate it with a possible cause you should start thinking 'neck' and 'back'. Have you ever had issues involving vertebrae or disks? Have you ever had a medical professional show you a plastic model of the backbone and point out where the discs lie and how the spinal nerves branch out? If so, there is a very good chance that your CPS could be due to a spinal cord issue.

And it does not have to have been recent. CPS does not always occur soon after the triggering cause. It has been known to happen quite a long time later. Maybe even a year, maybe more. So, you might have to think back, carefully. Plus, it might not have been that serious. You may have got over 'it' quite quickly and thought you were out of the woods. Then, out of the blue, you start getting these strange pains and weird sensations – possibly not that severely to begin with. But, it builds up progressively. This, alas, is another nasty aspect of CPS. It can strike without warning, long after the initial condition that disrupted the central nervous system.

EPILEPSY

Pain, let alone CPS, is not something often associated with epilepsy. A quick search on the Internet will show that there are quite a few epilepsy sufferers (or caregivers) inquiring as to whether pain is something that is to be expected. Interestingly pain, burning sensations, etc., are not listed by the '*Epilepsy Foundation*' in the section '*Impact*' that deals with the other problems that can occur following a seizure. This '*Impact*' section, however, mentions: depression, anxiety, mood changes, sleep disorders, '*not doing well*' and '*other illnesses*'.

The likes of WebMD and the Mayo Clinic in their discussions of epilepsy also mention the emotional issues, but not the pain. Thus, the connection between epilepsy and CPS is invariably only highlighted in documentation related to CPS.

That epilepsy could cause CPS should not be an issue of doubt or debate.

That the seizures associated with epilepsy are due to a disruption of the brain's electrical activity is widely understood and believed. WebMd states it simply as: *"Epilepsy is a disorder of the brain's electrical system"*. The Mayo Clinic, in its '*Overview*' of the condition, starts off by stating that: *"Epilepsy is a central nervous system disorder (neurological disorder) in which nerve cell activity in the brain becomes disrupted, causing seizures …"*.

As should be very clear by now any CNS disorder can result in CPS. Thus, it should not be surprising that epilepsy could result in CPS.

Epilepsy, furthermore, can be caused by head injuries, strokes, brain tumors and meningitis – all of which are also directly associated with CPS. So, there is even the chance that CPS was caused by something that happened prior to epilepsy.

A research study in 2014 showed that more than a quarter of patients with epilepsy are prescribed opioids for pain. Based on this, one could conclude that 'pain' is more common among epilepsy sufferers than in the general population at large.

PARKINSON'S DISEASE

Over 10 million people worldwide are believed to suffer from the movement-related issues associated with Parkinson's. A million or more of them are in the U.S. Of late the diagnosis rate is around 60,000 Americans per year. It is also appreciated that there are probably tens of thousands of instances worldwide (thousands of these in the U.S.) that still go undetected and undiagnosed.

The condition is named after **James Parkinson** [1755 to 1824], a British surgeon who was also active in medical chemistry, fossil hunting, geology and politics. In 1817 he published '*An Essay on the Shaking Palsy*' – the first scientific description of this long-term, progressively worsening disorder. The term "Parkinson's Disease" was coined in the late 1860s by the French neurologist, **Jean-Martin Charcot**, credited as being '*the founder of modern neurology*'. [Neurology is the branch of medicine related to nervous system disorders; a neurologist, a doctor specializing in neurology.]

As is the case with epilepsy, pain is not something often mentioned in the context of Parkinson's. The "*Parkinson's Disease Foundation*", however, has an article from 2005, written by a specialist from Columbia University, entitled "*Pain in Parkinson's Disease*". The third sentence of this article is as follows: "*And yet, when carefully questioned, more than half of all people with Parkinson's disease say that they have experienced painful symptoms and various forms of physical discomfort"*. More than half!

Per this article the symptoms most experienced are: aching, stiffness, numbness and tingling. These are, of course, some of the hallmarks of CPS. This article then goes onto say that in a few instances the pain and discomfort could be so severe that it overshadows the other problems arising from Parkinson's.

Parkinson's is defined as a long-term, progressive and irreversible disorder of the central nervous system that primarily impacts bodily movement. So, it is another CNS disorder – and hence the inevitable link to Central Pain Syndrome. As with so many CNS-related conditions there is, as yet, no known cure for Parkinson's.

Parkinson's usually strikes those who are over 60, affecting about 1% of this aging population. An early onset version can inflict those in their 40s and 50s; about 4% of Parkinson's sufferers diagnosed as such before they reach 50. The chances of getting Parkinson's does increase with age.

There is no specific test, e.g., blood test or scan, to conclusively determine Parkinson's. It is diagnosed through the presence of telltale symptoms.

In marked contrast to fibromyalgia and MS, significantly more males than females contract Parkinson's.

While the oft stated claim is *"you die with Parkinson's disease, not from it"*, it is also not unusual to find a '*between 7 to 14 years*' or '*an average of 16 years*' life expectancy quoted for this disease – this time period measured from the onset of the symptoms. These deaths are typically attributed to complications arising from Parkinson's such as swallowing difficulties or a heightened susceptibility for catching pneumonia.

OTHER CAUSES

The causes listed at the start of this chapter are considered, at present, to be the major (and best understood) triggers of CPS. But, there can be other causes as well. In essence any condition that *compromises* the brain or the nervous system, or *damages* the insulation that protects nerves (as in MS), can result in CPS – at some point down the road. In this context the nerve damage can extend beyond that of the central nervous system.

So, while the major causes of CPS are invariably associated with violations to the central nervous system, it is indeed possible to get CPS from nerve damage that occurs further out in the body.

The 'Central Pain Syndrome Foundation' has a list of *less common causes* of CPS which include (in alphabetical order):

o   AIDS, especially end-stage

o   Arachnoiditis

o   Arteriovenous malformation

o   Cauda equina syndrome

o   Cervical myelopathy

o   Charcot-Marie-Tooth disease

o   Chemical toxicity

o   Cluster headaches

o   Gunshot wounds

o   Lead neuropathy

o   Meralgia paresthetica

o   Mercury toxicity

o   Myelomalacia

o   Neurofibromatosis

o   *Polio*

o   Posterior myelitis

o   Prion disorders

o   Radiation exposure

o   Reflex sympathetic dystrophy syndrome

o   Spinal cord infarction

o   Syringomyelia

o   Tethered cord syndrome

o   Transverse myelitis

o   Vascular malformation

o   Vitamin B-12 deficiency

And this list is not meant to be complete either.

Charcot-Marie-Tooth disease is not a dental condition! It is named after three neurologists, the last, Dr. Howard Henry Tooth (of Britain). 'Charcot', the first mentioned, is the same Jean-Martin Charcot, 'the founder of modern neurology', that gave us the name "Parkinson's

Disease". Charcot-Marie-Tooth disease is a group of *inherited* disorders of the *peripheral nervous system.* So, this is an example of CPS symptoms being triggered by a disorder further downstream from the brain/spinal cord.

Vitamin B-12 deficiency is known to cause nerve-related issues leading to symptoms associated with CPS – i.e., numbness, weird sensations, tingling and weakness, especially in one's legs, feet or hands. It can also cause psychological issues such as depression, confusion, memory loss and mood changes. Vitamin B-12 deficiency, often due to dietary habits, is easy enough to detect (with a simple blood test), and, in the majority of cases, to treat (with a modified diet, multivitamins or supplements). The deficiency can be prevented and corrected – worst case with weekly Vitamin B-12 injections. Thus, *unlike with CPS in general*, CPS-like symptoms due to a Vitamin B-12 deficiency could be cured or greatly minimized. *[Refer to the 'Glossary' for descriptions of the other terms.]*

Diabetes

Note that diabetes has not been mentioned as either a major or 'less common' cause. This is not an oversight, bias or prejudice. Diabetes is always conspicuous by its absence in discussions to do with CPS. Nerve pain, however, is a common side-effect of diabetes, affecting at least 50% of diabetics. There is even a (fairly well known) name for it: *diabetic peripheral neuropathy* – sometimes referred to just as *diabetic neuropathy or peripheral neuropathy.*

Neuropathy means that it is a nerve-related disease. ['*Neuro*', from the Greek, denoting that it relates to nerves or the nervous system, and '*pathy*', also from Greek, indicating that it is a disease or suffering.]

There are *three* different types of nerve damage associated with diabetic neuropathy. These are as follows. Damage to nerves that control muscle movement -- *motor neuropathy*. Damage to nerves that provide the sensations of touch and feeling – *sensory neuropathy*. Damage to nerves that manage vital bodily functions such as: heart rate, blood pressure, body temperature, waste disposal and digestion – *autonomic neuropathy*.

If there is damage to both motor and sensory nerves it is called *sensorimotor neuropathy*, while **polyneuropathy** is used to describe widespread nerve damage.

The pain associated with diabetic neuropathy is often extreme, relentless, persistent and hard to control. It may have started as a tingling that soon progressed to numbness and pain. Nerve damage to the feet is particularly prevalent, and can lead to severe complications unless adequately treated.

There is obviously some commonality between the symptoms of diabetic neuropathy and CPS.

There appears to be two reasons as to why diabetic neuropathy is excluded as a cause of CPS. The first being that it is very much a *peripheral* neuropathy – as indicated by its name. Though there are exceptions, such as Charcot-Marie-Tooth disease, CPS, by and large, per the '*central*' in its name, is attributed to central nervous system disorders.

The second reason for its exclusion, most likely has to do with the fact that diabetic peripheral neuropathy is a well-defined, and well dealt with, condition in its own right. The care and treatment for it is handled routinely as a part of the standard diabetes management protocols. Suffice to say that many of the treatment options for diabetic neuropathy are the same as those for CPS. A good example of this is *Lyrica* (pregabalin), a drug manufactured by Pfizer. Though initially developed as an anti-epileptic drug, it is now widely used to treat Fibromyalgia, diabetic nerve pain, spinal cord injury nerve pain and CPS. *[See an advertisement below.]*

When A Cause Is Not Obvious

More often than not the probable cause of CPS does not remain a mystery for long.

If a stroke, MS, Parkinson's or such has already been determined, it is unlikely that doctors will look any further – though there could also be other contributing factors. If it is not one of these 'biggies' it could likely be traced back to a head injury, a damaged spinal disc, an infection (e.g., some form of encephalitis), back surgery, whiplash, or an aneurysm. Failing that, some initial tests, such as an MRI or a battery of blood tests, might uncover a cause (unwelcome though it may be) – a tumor, an infection, spinal column deterioration, etc.

All this said, there can still be some instances when the possible cause for the CPS continues to remain elusive. The growing trend of late appears to be for doctors, in such cases, to start *treating the symptoms*, without always feeling that they have to first identify a specific cause – provided, of course, that they have eliminated all of the potentially harmful 'biggies' (e.g., undetected aneurysm, tumors, onset of MS or even diabetes).

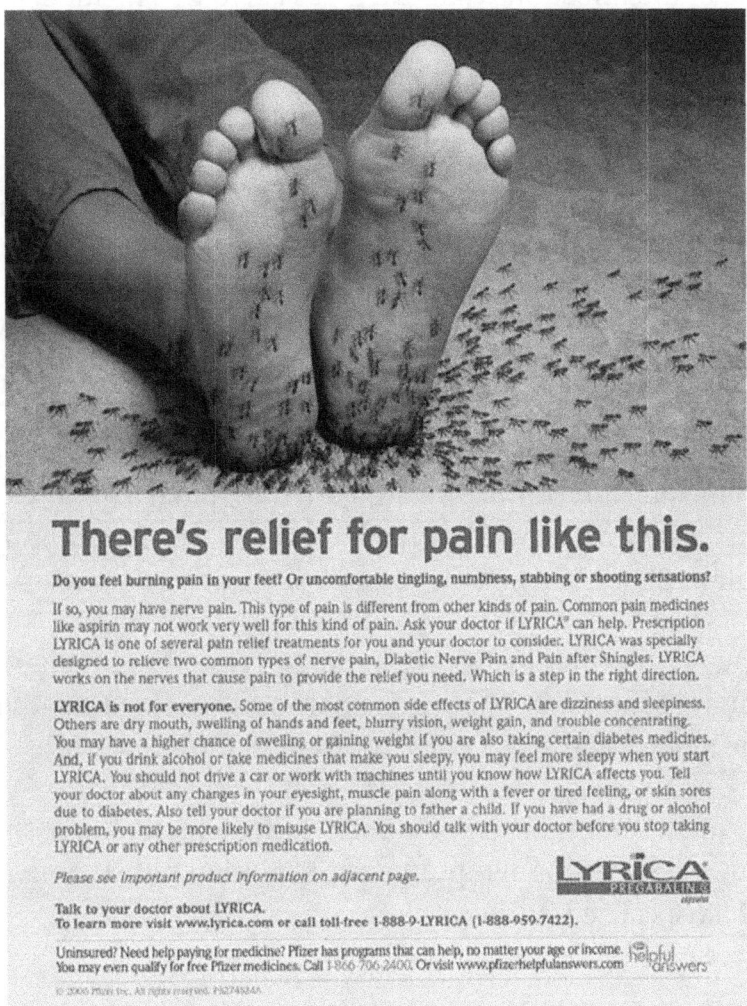

An advertisement for Pfizer's *Lyrica* pain medication.

TAKEAWAYS:
CHAPTER 3 – POSSIBLE CAUSES

ം CPS is always an unexpected consequence of something that happened *previously* to disrupt the normal workings of the central nervous system (CNS), i.e., brain, brain stem and spinal cord.

ം The most common causes that can eventually lead to CPS *include*: stroke, multiple sclerosis (MS), head/spinal cord injuries, tumors/cancer in or around the brain/spinal column, epilepsy, procedures/surgeries, Parkinson's disease, aneurysms and CNS-related infections.

ം *Some* of the infections that can give rise to CPS include: meningitis, shingles, late stage Lyme disease, tuberculosis, most types of encephalitis, Guillain–Barré syndrome, malaria, etc.

ം ~10% of stroke patients, at least 20% of those with MS, and possibly half of those with Parkinson's, end up having the symptoms of CPS.

ം CPS may also be due to other less common causes, a few of them more related to the *peripheral*, as opposed to central, nervous system.

ം Any mishap or trauma related to the spinal column (including surgeries or procedures), even if it was quite a '*longtime ago*', could result in CPS.

ം Diabetic neuropathy, though nerve-related and sharing some common symptoms, is not considered as causing CPS – though the same medication, e.g., *Lyrica,* is often used to treat both.

ം If a cause cannot be readily determined, doctors, per the current norm, will treat the symptoms of CPS without obsessing as to what may have caused its onset.

4.
PAIN &
THE BRAIN

Pain with Central Pain Syndrome is widespread and varied. That is a defining characteristic of CPS. *In reality, however,* **all this pain***, in all its forms, is all being felt* **in the brain** *– and nowhere else!*

You read that right.

All pain is in the brain.

But, this has <u>NOTHING</u> to do with CPS.

Everybody, *whether they have CPS or not,* can only feel pain in their brain. That is an inescapable fact of life, all to do with the way the human body works. The brain is the only organ in our body capable of *creating* pain. The brain, clever as it is, makes us feel that pain where we think it is coming from. It is like ventriloquism, where a ventriloquist makes their voice appear to be coming from somewhere else. The pain is being *felt* in the brain, but the brain makes it feel like it is coming from somewhere else.

All of this is independent of whether you have CPS or not. *That is always important to keep in mind.*

There are, however, **three things different for those with CPS.**

One of these is that the brain unintentionally amplifies all of its responses to pain. This is what often gets described as the: *"volume being turned up on the body's pain system"*, or the *hypersensitivity* to pain. So, what pre-CPS may have felt like a '4' on the pain scale now feels like a '7'. That is a problem. The medical term for it is *Hyperalgesia* – *'algesia'* being the Greek for 'pain'. [The *'algia'*, in Fibromyalgia, is Latin for pain.]

This pain-amplification is definitely a part of the CPS 'disorder'. One of the things that has gone awry within the CNS. It is *thought* to be due to the brain being overwhelmed by the amount of pain-related processing it has *had to do,* over time, in the case of CPS sufferers.

But, then there is a second factor that makes this worse. When you have CPS, the brain receives *confusing*, and sometimes *downright false*, pain signals via the spinal cord and the brain stem. The brain has no way of knowing that these pain signals are 'unnatural' or invalid. It treats them the same way as genuine pain signals. However, since the *'volume is already turned up'* the pain is worse. So, yes, with CPS two things definitely out of the ordinary are already taking place when it comes to pain: confusing/invalid pain signals plus the *hypersensitivity*.

There is a belief that this *over-amplification* of pain starts because the brain is getting all these confusing/invalid pain signals. These 'bogus' pain signals appear to send the brain's pain management system into a frenzy. Makes it go haywire. *This pain-amplification is definitely a part of CPS*. And it will **_NOT_** be limited to just the CPS-related pain. It will apply to **_ALL_** pain.

A double-whammy already. And, alas, it gets worse!

How we deal with pain is influenced by our emotional state of mind. That is well known and understood. When we are emotionally distressed pain always seems worse and more upsetting. That in turn, can further amplify the brain's response to pain.

As such, the pain-volume gets cranked up further when we are distressed.

The added pain causes MORE emotional distress ... which in turn makes you <u>even more</u> sensitive to pain.

This cranks up the pain-volume *another notch – to **<u>ALL pain</u>***.

You get the picture?

It is a vicious cycle.

*It is now a **triple whammy**.*

An unwelcome trifecta of pain.

So, yes, with CPS *three things*, out of the ordinary, are happening – all within the brain. The brain is receiving 'bad' pain signals, and the brain is overreacting to them. The added pain causes added emotional distress (i.e., depression and anxiety) which in turn amplifies the pain ... causing more emotional distress, which in turn ...

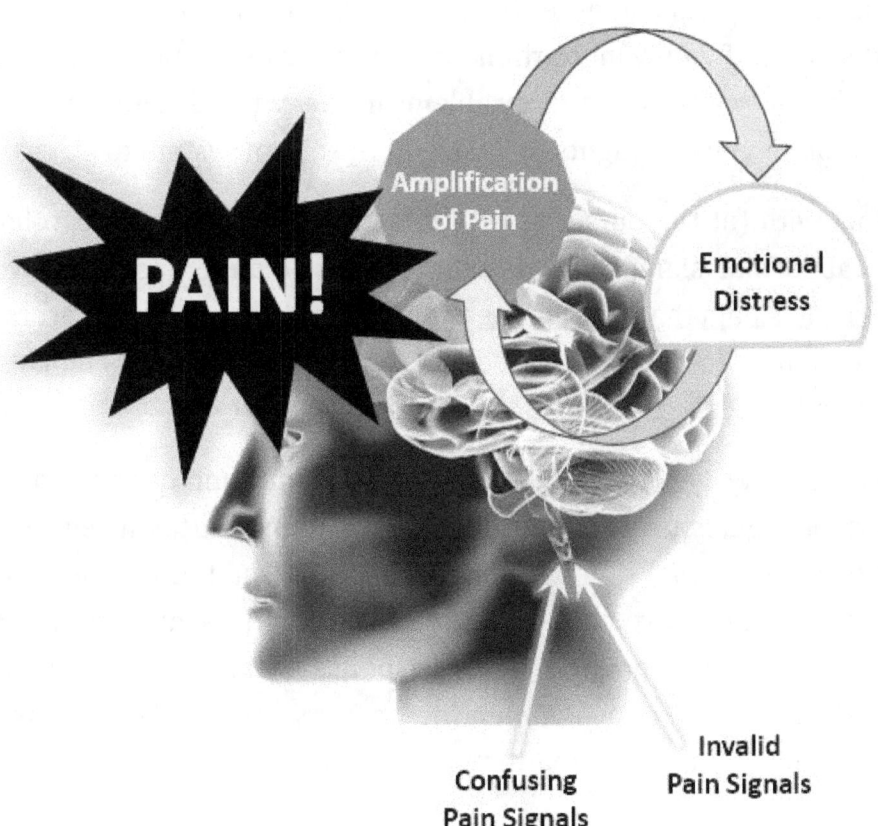

Hence, the overall exaggerated pain of CPS. This is why it is considered a disorder of the central nervous system. It is the spinal cord, the brain stem and in the end, the brain *inadvertently* creating intense pain – when, in reality, the pain should not be as such.

A QUICK CPS PERSPECTIVE
OF THE PAIN-BRAIN CONNECTION

If you were not already aware of this, being told that *'all pain is in the brain'*, understandably, comes as quite a shock – possibly even an affront.

There is nothing one can do about the pain-brain connection.

It is how the human body functions – how our entire nervous system and brain are '*hardwired*' to work.

The wiring metaphor is useful. CPS is when the body's wiring harness, i.e., the nervous system, starts to malfunction – causing the brain, the body's inbuilt, all-powerful computer (so to speak), to continually get all sorts of weird signals. If you want to think of it in terms of wiring in a car, CPS is when short-circuits and other problems in the wiring harness causes the horn to blare, the headlights to flash and the alarm system to go crazy.

To start with (at the outset of CPS) the brain will do its best to handle these 'abnormal' signals in a normal, 'orderly' manner. So, there will be pain – be it is pain that has not been exaggerated. Some CPS sufferers may be able to think back to that phase. There was pain, but it was much more muted and easier to deal with.

It appears, however, that over time the frequency and quantity of these 'abnormal' signals drive the brain to distraction. *That is when the pain amplification sets in.* From then on it is downhill, all the way. Not only is the brain getting more pain signals than normal (because the wiring is damaged) it is also amplifying its response to all the pain signals it receives. *It is a double whammy.* Now factor in the emotional distress, which further compounds matters. But, that is, alas, what is happening.

That all pain is in the brain, *CPS or otherwise*, sometimes gets seen as: *'the pain is really all in your head'*. This is upsetting to many. They feel that this makes it sound as if their pain is not real. Not so. **The pain is real, very real**. It is just happening within the brain – and 'that', i.e., that it is happening in the brain, has nothing, whatsoever, to do with CPS.

Yes, the notion that pain is *always* in the brain rather than where you are experiencing it can be confusing, galling and frustrating. But, there is nothing you, or anybody else, can do about it.

You have heard the claim: *'there is no gain without pain'*.

Well, it is also true that: *'there is no pain without brain'*!

So, that is, alack, the dilemma faced by those with CPS. Your central nervous system is conspiring against you. You can't help it. Something, somewhere went wrong causing this malfunctioning of the CNS. It is like any other irreversible condition. It is a shame, it is unfortunate, it is upsetting, it is frustrating, it is depressing – but, it has happened, and it is unlikely to ever fully go away.

That the pain is in the brain, by itself, is NOT something worth railing about. *That part is independent of CPS*. Don't get bent out of shape that the pain is in your head. That is normal. All pain is *created* in your brain.

What is abnormal are the 'incorrect' pain signals and the brain's hypersensitivity to all pain. So, it is really important to be clear about this – and to keep it in perspective. That pain is in your head is normal and natural. You can't change that part. So, you have to learn to live with that, i.e., *'all pain is really all in your head'*. PERIOD.

THE BASICS OF THE PAIN-BRAIN CONNECTION

If this is the first time you have heard of the pain-brain connection, let me, please, make a suggestion. If you have access to the Internet do a search on *"pain and the brain"* as well as *"all pain is in the brain"*. That way you can get a ton of information from different viewpoints (from some credible sources), and come to realize that this 'pain-brain connection' is not something new -- or just made up to infuriate CPS sufferers.

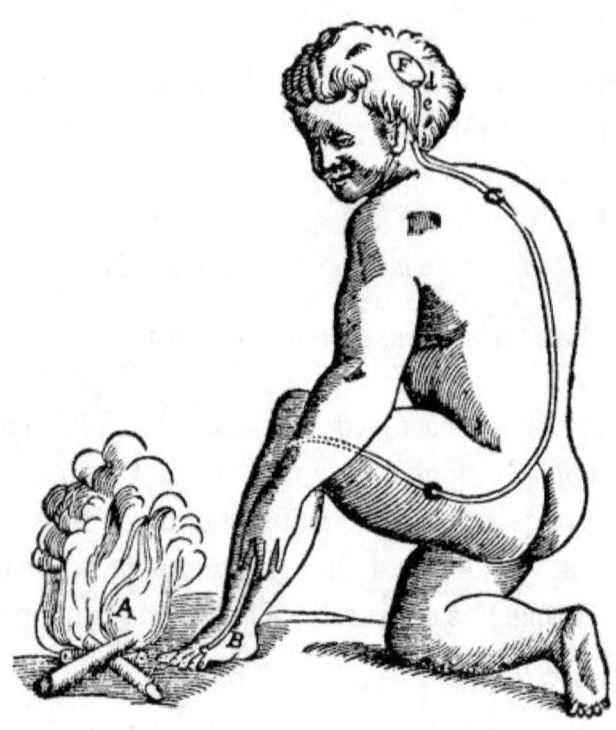

An illustration, related to pain, from 1664, in the book
'*Traite de l'homme*' (Treatise of Man), by René Descartes,
the French philosopher considered to be the
father of modern western philosophy, showing that
the pain-brain connection has been known
for over 350 years.

I really would like you to do this research. When you do, you should be able to find entries such as: '*Pain in the Brain*', '*Pain is in the Brain*', '*Pain Signals to the Brain from the Spine*', '*Pain Really is all in Your Head And Emotions Controls Intensity*', '*Understanding the Brain is the Key to Being Pain-Free*', and '*How the Brain Interprets Pain and How to Get Relief*', etc. Always consider the source and just focus on the ones that appear to be from credible sources. There is much you can learn.

I am not going to spend too much time trying to explain the intricacies of all that is involved. It can very quickly get very technical and complex. You end up having to start talking about the *amygdala region* of the brain (that handles pain and emotion) or *neurotransmitter receptors* (a.k.a. *neuroreceptors*), that perform complex chemical processes as the brain handles sensory signals. That is a level of detail that is just overwhelming. The goal here is to keep it simple, factual, on-point, easy to understand – and *relevant to CPS*.

It Is All About Perception

Pain starts off as a *sensation*. Any sensation is a *stimulation* on or within the body that causes 'sensory nerves' to send *sensory information* to the brain via the spinal cord. How the brain interprets and reacts to sensory information is called *perception.*

So, pain starts off as a sensation and then becomes a perception when the brain processes the sensory information.

All of this brain activity, including the interpretation of the sensory information and the creation of the perception, is achieved by means of chemical and electrical interactions (within the brain).

Sight, sound, smell, taste, balance, feeling of temperature and sense of motion are also *all sensations* that have to be perceived by the brain. *So, it all 'being in the brain' is by no means limited just to pain.*

These words you are reading are not being formed – let alone recognized and interpreted – by your eyes. The eyes just act as focusing lenses and light/dark/color detecting optical sensors. It is the brain that *sees* the sensory information produced by the eyes. It is said that at least two-thirds of the brain is devoted to providing sight. That should show how central the brain is when it comes to making sensory information meaningful.

That we only 'see' via the brain is why there can be optical illusions and why we can enjoy animated cartoons such as the timeless classics from Disney. Animation, even with today's sophisticated computer generated imagery, is still achieved by a series of still images – with small differences in where objects appear in each image. The smooth motion we see is *created in our brain* when we are shown those still images in rapid succession.

And it is not just sight. Sound, smell and taste are also all in the brain. We don't actually hear things within our ears. The sound is created in the brain. The ears just send detailed information about the vibrations they are detecting to the brain. The brain synthesizes that information to create the appropriate sounds. That people can lose their sense of smell, taste or both as a result of a brain injury is well known and documented. Yet another example of how we are so dependent on the brain for all of our sensory experiences.

The Perception Of Pain

The perception of pain, *independent of CPS*, varies, quite a bit, from person to person. It can also vary within a person at *different times* – depending on their emotional state. The more emotionally distressed you are, the greater your inclination to feel more pain. And that as we have already seen is a cruel, vicious cycle.

The perception of pain cannot be generalized. No two people are likely to perceive pain in exactly the same way. The claim *'I feel your pain'* is rarely, if ever, true. A claim, however, of '*I have a high tolerance to pain*' or '*I used to have a high tolerance of pain, but not anymore*' is probably very true. That is about perception, i.e., one's ability to control and alter the feeling of pain. Yes, the ability to control/alter the feeling of pain, i.e., modulating pain, becomes a *challenge with CPS*. That is a given.

Pain is one of the body's most important defense mechanisms. It tells us when something bad has happened to the body. If we hit our head, burn a finger, bang our foot or twist an ankle, the pain (perceived in the brain) tells us that something needs our immediate attention. This is also the case with pain associated with an infection, a growth or internal bleeding. It is to tell us that something is wrong and needs attention.

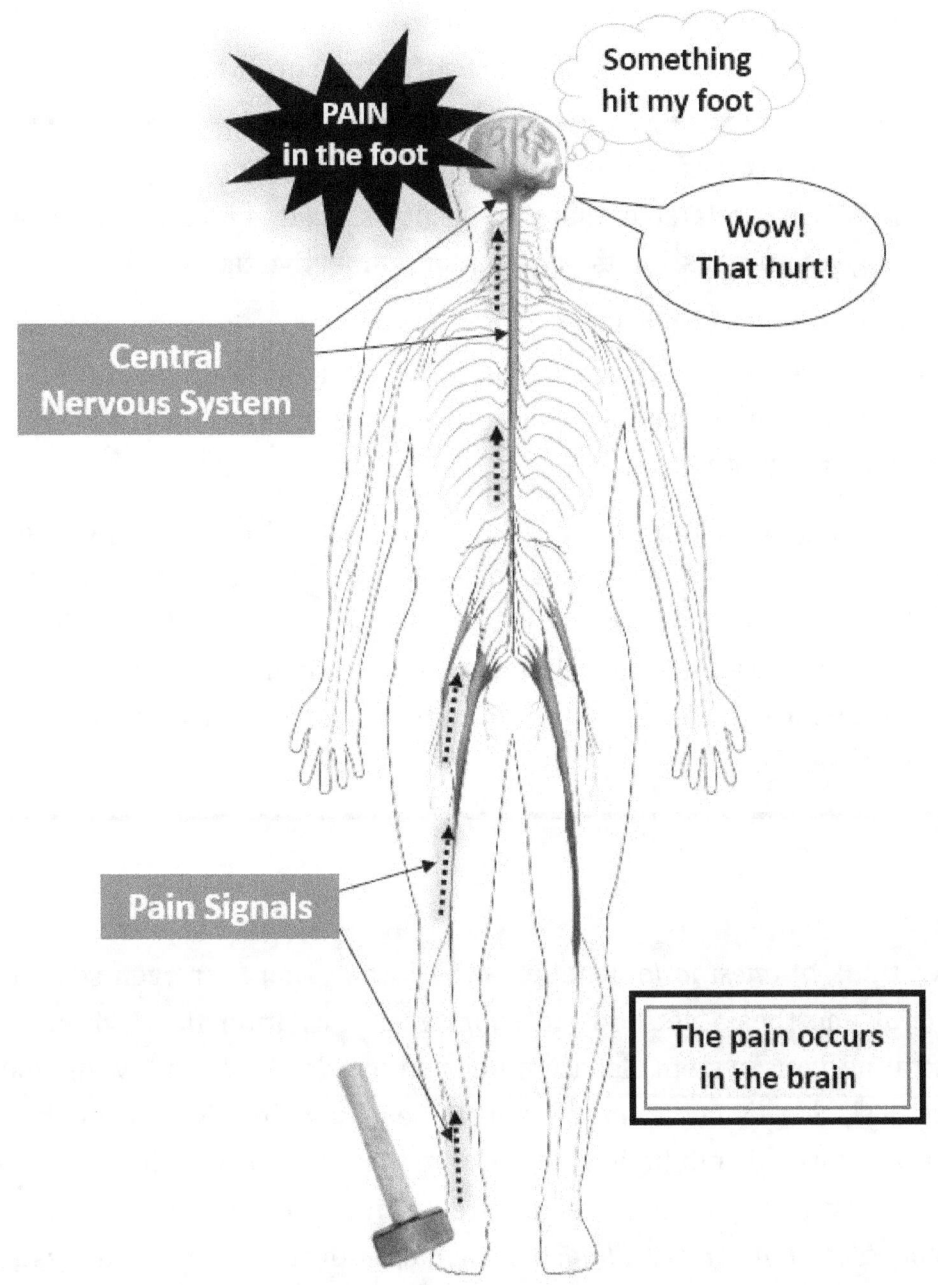

Without pain we could keep on getting in harm's way. There are some people that feel no pain – because of a defect in their CNS. Not being able to perceive pain is not the blessing you would initially think. These folks have to go through life being extremely careful. They could quite literally toast their hand on a hot surface and not know about it. The smell of burning flesh could be their first intimation – and that is not good.

So, pain has a purpose. It is pain *due to a fault in the central nervous system*, as is the case with CPS, that is a tiresome problem.

In chapter 1 it was said that **fibromyalgia** is *no longer* considered to be arthritis-related in that there is **_no_** associated inflammation or damage to muscles, joints, tendons, or connective tissue!

The pain being experienced is not caused by an inflammation or injury. *Well, ditto in the case of CPS*. The pain, in both instances, is due to the brain receiving invalid pain signals as opposed to any real inflammation or injury.

So, hoping to reduce or stop the pain by treating the supposed inflammation or injury is **not** going to help. This, understandably, drives some CPS sufferers to distraction – and beyond. If the pain is coming from a joint or muscle, and you can actually feel it there, why can't it be treated at the source? And that, alas and alack, is the crux and curse of CPS.

Anesthesia & Opioids

Now, think of *anesthesia*, whether it be local, general or even sedation. General anesthesia sets out to *suppress* information flow within the central nervous system. Sedation does so to a lesser extent, while local anesthesia *blocks nerve impulses* from reaching the CNS. All of this is achieved through modifying *chemical activity* within the CNS which in turn affect the way electrical signals flow within nerves. So, anesthesia is all about '*blocking and tackling*' pain signals at the central nervous system level, through chemical intervention. This *interferes with the perception of pain* by the brain. That is how the pain minimization is realized.

Opioids (e.g., oxycodone, methadone, morphine), often used to treat CPS, contrary to what some may swear by, do not work by removing (or treating) the cause of pain. Instead, they work by reducing the *perception of pain* <u>within the brain</u> -- and at the same time encouraging the brain to produce a sense of well-being and pleasure. This is the so called *opioid euphoria*. Opioids achieve their goal by stimulating the release of natural brain chemicals – in particular **endorphins** (that reduce pain) and **dopamine** (the body's feel-good chemical).

There are two things, however, that you should note when it comes to opioids. The first is that they work purely by altering brain chemistry. That is vital to remember. Therefore, opioids do not reduce the intensity level or volume of pain signals reaching the brain. They just try to get the brain to react less to the pain and trick the brain into believing life is indeed good. The second thing is not to let the '*they trigger the release of **natural** brain chemicals*' statement lead you astray. The problem is that the brain is being tricked into releasing these chemicals.

Tricking the brain can lead both to the over stimulation of the pain management system, as well as for the brain to keep on expecting '*more of the same*' since it appeared to have been a 'good thing'. The overstimulation can lead to *opioid-induced hyperalgesia* (the hypersensitivity to pain) while the '*more of the same*' is what causes dependence/addiction.

The opioid-induced hyperalgesia should be of particular concern to those with CPS. Hyperalgesia, outside of opioid use, is one of the biggest problems in CPS – as we have already seen. Prolonged opioid use to deal with CPS can add a whole new dimension of hyperalgesia to what was already there to begin with! That is the problem, in a nutshell.

Yes, you can seriously compound the *hyperalgesia* problem with opioids – and that is before you run into any dependency issues. And remember that hyperalgesia applies to **<u>ALL pain</u>**, not just to those related to-CPS. So everything is more painful!

Mind Over Matter

'*Mind over matter*', in the context of pain, if you hadn't already thought of it, is another compelling example of the pain-brain connection. Mind over matter takes the notion of pain tolerance to a whole new, and often an incredibly impressive, level.

You no doubt have heard the stories of folks that have had major operations without anesthetics. Then there are all those amazing pain defying feats associated with Indian yogis and religious devotees. [*Refer to the picture below.*] If you would like to learn more, Google: '*Hindu cheek piercing*', '*Hindu pain devotion*' and '*Hindu firewalking*'. And while you are at it, you might as well also check '*mind over matter controlling pain*'.

The featured theme of the December 2016 issue of the venerable '*National Geographic*' magazine was '*The Healing Power of Faith*'. You may want to try and get a copy of this article online or from a library. It offers some highly illuminating insights as to the power of mind over matter, as well as the *placebo effect* (discussed below).

This article starts off with the story of a German man, in his early 60s, who completed a 70-mile pilgrimage, on foot, despite *the pain* from a broken heel that he had recently suffered. His desire to undertake and complete the pilgrimage somehow managed to let him endure and overcome the pain – though he wasn't sure at the start whether he would be able to walk that far. Just another data point when it comes to the possibility of modulating (i.e., controlling/modifying/varying) pain via the power of thought and belief – where this 'belief' is not specific to any one religion.

Obviously, modulating pain via mind over matter is not something that applies to all. If it was, the worldwide pain care industry would not be so enormously huge and you would not be reading this book! For CPS sufferers, however, the potential of mind over matter, regarding pain, should be a goal, an inspiration – something worth striving for.

Meditation and yoga do fall into the realm of mind over matter. Their power to help cope with pain is well publicized. Meditation, in particular, is easy enough to do. Now that you are familiar with the pain-brain connection you must be able to see how meditation, which is all in the mind, might help manage pain.

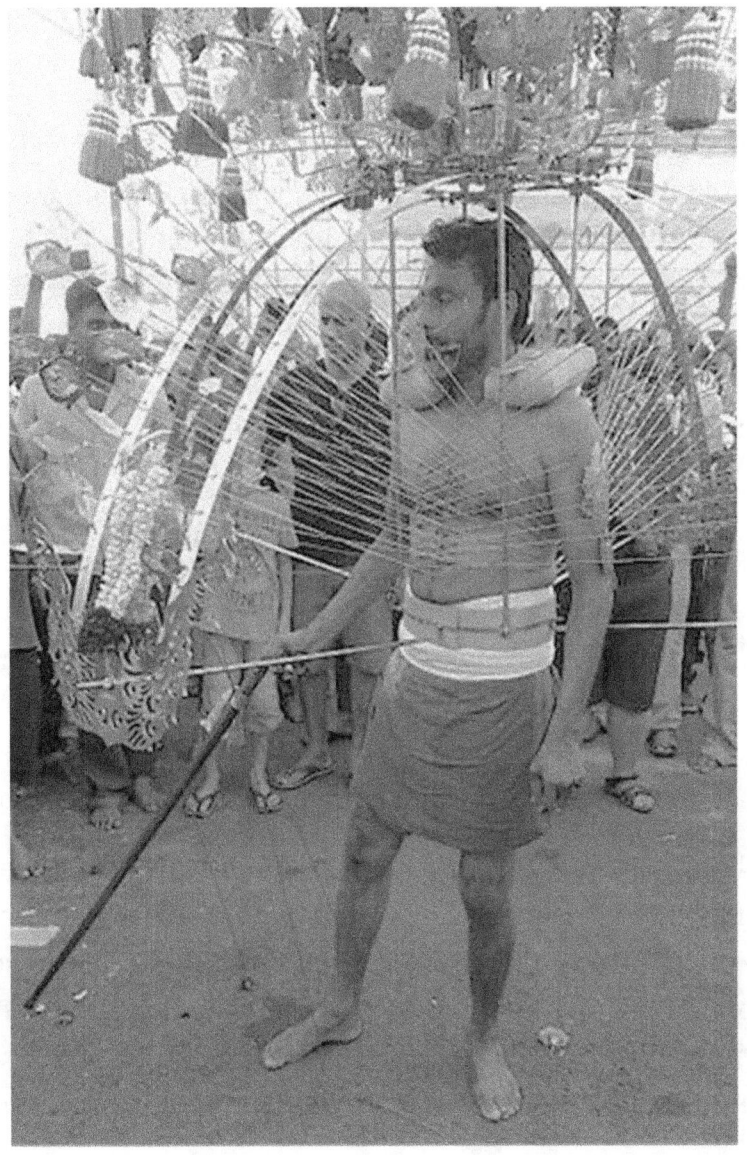

Ceremonial piercing of the skin and other pain-related practices
for religious purposes – in this case an example of the Hindu
Kavadi Attam which may involve up to 108 piercings.

From: Wikipedia

Yes, some forms of meditation will trigger the release of *endorphins*,
dopamine and other *natural brain chemicals* without the help of any
drugs. Triggering the release of these chemicals, albeit possibly in smaller
doses, through meditation and yoga, is seen by most as being

considerably more desirable than a reliance on drugs – particularly opioids.

I, the author of this book, believe in, and promote, a very concentrated form of meditation referred to as '*Brain Meditation*'. 'Brain meditation' is meant to be done in background mode, while you proceed with your normal, day-to-day life. The very concentrated nature of it is geared to stimulate *good* brain chemical activity with minimal effort. It is a form of meditation that could help many with CPS – per the accepted beliefs of mind over matter when it comes to pain modulation.

The Placebo Effect

'*Placebo*' is from the Latin for '*I please*'. It is a pill, a potion, an injection, an inhalant, a procedure or a treatment with **no** medicinal value. It is a '*fake*' medicinal treatment masquerading as something very real, with the power to cure. A placebo is always meant to be totally harmless with no active ingredients that could cause any adverse reactions. Placebos, however, are not meant to do what they are *said to be* capable of doing.

Placebos have to be used in drug evaluations and approvals to determine the true effectiveness of a new drug. One controlled group is given the real drug/treatment while another is given a placebo under the guise that it is the real thing. Then the results from the two groups are compared. Ideally the group that got the real drug/treatment should have exhibited a considerably higher success rate than those that got the placebo.

Placebo testing of drugs invariably comes up with some intriguing results. The success rate within the placebo control group is rarely, if ever, zero. In the case of Viagra (for ED) 11% of those that were given the placebo claimed it had worked just as expected. While the effectiveness was two to three times greater among those given the real thing, the placebo results do give one pause for thought.

In the case of opioids, there have been some remarkable results attributed to the placebo effect. A much quoted, landmark study was done in 1978 by University of California (San Francisco) rheumatologist Jon Levine and neurologist Howard Fields on patients who underwent wisdom tooth extraction. Many of those that were given an injection of saline solution claimed they experienced a reduction in pain.

Interestingly the placebo effect with opioids is easy to understand and well known among the medical community. It all has to do with the brains built in 'reward mechanism' and *expectations*. The *belief* that one is getting powerful pain relieving medication triggers the release of endorphins – the body's natural pain medication.

Scientists now consider the supposed benefits of both acupuncture and cupping (much publicized by the U.S. swim team at the 2016 Olympics) to be due to the placebo effect – particularly when it comes to the claims of long-term relief.

The December 2016 '*National Geographic*' article '*The Healing Power of Faith*', referenced above, includes a very illuminating case of a U.S. male, in his 40s, who was suffering from early onset Parkinson's disease. In 2011 he opted to undergo an experimental gene therapy that appeared to have been rather successful when tested on monkeys. Two holes were cut in his skull and the drug was injected directly into his brain – one injection for each hemisphere of his brain.

His recovery following this procedure was miraculous. It appeared that Parkinson's had not just been slowed down or halted – it had been reversed. He was hardly exhibiting any symptoms of the disease.

Two years after he received his treatment it was announced that this gene therapy did not work! Further testing of the therapy was abandoned.

Sometime later, a doctor reexamining the miraculous recovery by this subject discovered something that (per the article) '*stopped her cold*'. Though they had drilled real holes in his skull, this lucky patient had not received the real drug. He had been injected with a placebo!

Doctors, at least in the U.S., per '*American Medical Association*' (AMA) guidelines, *cannot* prescribe placebos (outside of a clinical trial). U.S. doctors always must prescribe a drug or procedure that has some medicinal value; in the case of a drug it has to contain some active ingredients. Doctors, worldwide, however, are known to intentionally _hype_ the powers of drugs and procedures in the hope of gaining some placebo headwind. So, they might prescribe a less potent drug, with less harmful side effects, but make it sound as if it is much more powerful. The placebo effect has very few negative side effects! {Smile}

For those with CPS, the significance of the placebo effect is that it demonstrates, once again, the pain-brain connection – and the _possibility_ of gaining some solace through _mind over matter_. Enough said.

You have probably heard of _phantom limb pain_. This is the very real and sometimes extreme pain that some amputees feel in a limb that is no longer there. Phantom limb pain is a neuropathic pain – a pain caused by damage to or a dysfunction of the central nervous system. CPS is also a neuropathic pain.

In neither case, phantom limb pain or CPS, is anyone saying that the pain is phantom. **The pain is very real**. That is a given. The mystery is what is causing the brain to create that pain – other than it being due to a disorder of the central nervous system.

By now, given all that we have covered, you should have a fairly good grasp of how _vital it is to know and appreciate_ the brain-pain connection. The more you understand this connection the better it is for you when coping with CPS.

I will again stress that good information on '_all pain is in the brain_' is plentiful and readily available, especially on the Web. It is a topic, for obvious reasons, that has been much studied, for a long time. So, if you feel you would like to learn more, start with the Web or visit a library or bookstore. You can also, if possible, talk to a medical professional. Psychologists also know a lot about this topic. It is something they all have to learn about, in-depth. Many are reluctant to bring it up unless asked. So, go ahead – and ask.

There is also no shortage of information on the Web about the placebo effect, opioids, and phantom limb pain. It might interest you to discover that the U.S. Founding Father, Benjamin Franklin (of flying a kite during a thunder storm fame), in 1782, helped French King, Louis XIV, in uncovering a medical hoax – the so called '*animal magnetism cure*'. It was demonstrated to be nothing more than a placebo effect. What is sobering to realize is that this was over 200 years ago! As the French saying goes: *plus ça change, plus c'est la même chose* (the more it changes, the more it's the same thing).

The Brain Never Hurts!

This is the ultimate of ironies. Though it is the brain that creates pain, it is *NOT* possible for the brain itself to ever hurt! Why?

Because there are *no* pain sensation-related nerves in the brain itself.

So, the brain *never* receives any pain signals that says there is something wrong in the brain itself. Therefore, perceptions of pain, within the brain itself, never get generated.

However, the three-layer *membrane* that surrounds the brain does contain pain-sensing nerves as do some of the blood vessels feeding the brain. So, it is these nerves that can generate pain signals in the brain area. Typically, if there is something wrong within the brain, say bleeding or a tumor, pressure will be exerted on the surrounding membrane that will result in pain.

The tissue, i.e., the scalp, outside of the skull has pain sensing nerves, as do the back of the head and the neck. Any pain that we feel in our head could also be from these areas. Thus, a headache is usually due to pain sensations that originated in the forehead, the back of the head or the neck.

The statement '*my brain hurts*' is ambiguous. Your brain itself cannot hurt, but, then again, all the pain is, of course, coming from the brain. In the scheme of things this may appear a minor point, the splitting of hairs. Nonetheless, it is a point that has to be stressed in order to keep this pain discussion above-board and beyond contention.

**The Malfunctioning
'Check Engine' Light Analogy**

The only thing, in the whole car,
that is faulty is the 'Check Engine' <u>light</u>.

Repairing or replacing every other part in
the car will <u>not</u> turn off the light.

The only thing that has to be
fixed is the light itself
and, alas, it cannot be fixed!

THE CPS-RELATED IMPLICATIONS
OF THE PAIN-BRAIN CONNECTION

Knowing that all the pain of CPS is somewhere in the brain is of little comfort or consolation when you are in pain.

But, there are some real consequences to truly appreciating the pain-brain connection when dealing and coping with CPS.

Maybe this automotive analogy will drive the point home. CPS is the equivalent of the '*Check Engine*' **LIGHT** on a car malfunctioning – and, moreover, it being impossible to fix that malfunction. The light is ON, but it does not mean there is anything at all wrong in the car – other than the light! <u>You can replace every single component and probe in the car and the light will still remain on</u>.

That is the pain of CPS; the malfunctioning '*Check Engine*' light being the central nervous system. And, as you could in a car, you can't, unfortunately, just put a piece of duct tape over the light to hide it. But, that is what is really required: either the ability to replace the 'light' or being able to put a piece of duct tape over it. Hoping the light will finally turn off if yet one last tweak was done to the engine is but clutching at straws; just wishful thinking.

For a start, knowing the pain-brain connection will help when it comes to evaluating treatment options. Applying a topical cream to sooth a burning sensation on the arm is unlikely to be effective *when* the pain is due to an *invalid* pain signal. What you need to be looking for are treatments that somehow, in some way, block or modify the pain sensations flowing through the central nervous system, or alter the way the brain processes those sensations.

Recall what was said, in the previous section, about anesthesia. Anesthesia 'eliminates' pain by either suppressing the CNS or blocking pain signals from reaching the CNS. So, with CPS, you need to think along similar lines. As it happens one of the popular treatment options for CPS is a local anesthetic, **lidocaine**.

Lidocaine (also known as xylocaine and lignocaine) is a topical jelly or ointment. Lidocaine works by temporarily interfering with the *electrical impulses* used by nerves to transmit their sensory information. It manages to do so by changing sodium (i.e., salt) levels at nerve endings. This minimizes the nerves ability to transmit *any* signals. So, potential pain signals, real or invalid, are prevented from reaching the central nervous system. Bingo! And this what you should be seeking.

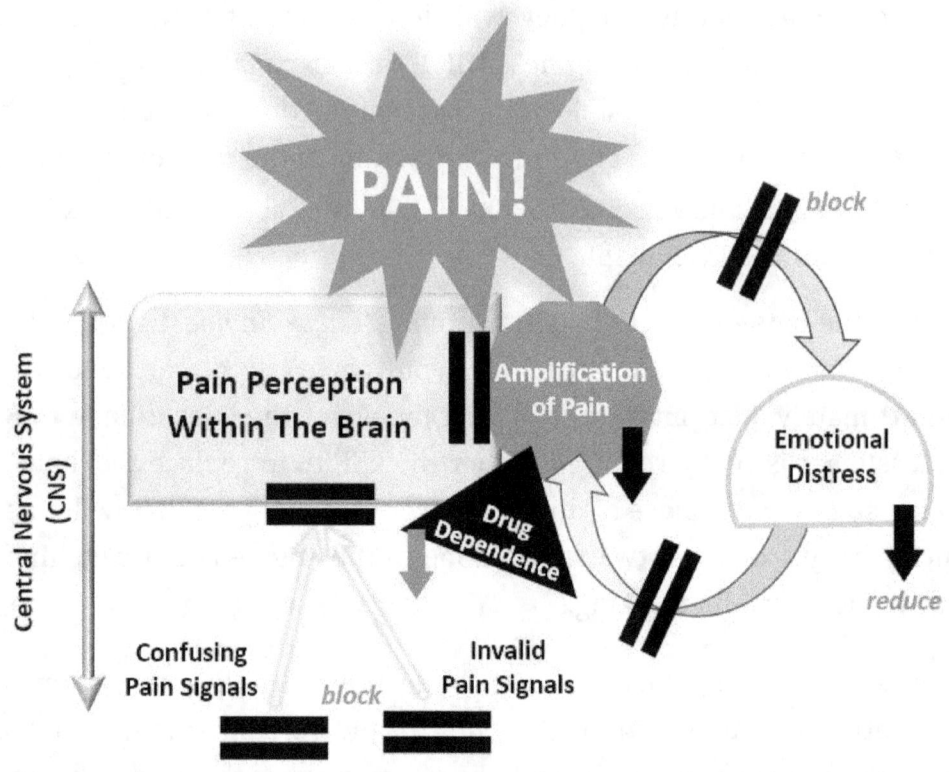

The <u>only</u> realistic options for reducing the pain of CPS.
But, this is easier said than done. And that is a problem.
However, trying to gain relief by attempting to tackle
the 'pain' elsewhere might not be effective.
It is the malfunctioning 'Check Engine' <u>light</u> dilemma.

If a treatment option does not seem to be targeted at the way the brain handles pain, or at suppressing/blocking pain at the CNS-level, you may want to really dig deep as to how it is supposed to work.

The tremendous possibilities of mind over matter, and the placebo effect, should never be underestimated. *Meditation* is an easy way to try and get some mind over matter benefits. You should now be able to see how anything that involves brain activity, in a concentrated manner, could touch upon the pain-brain connection. *Meditation is known to trigger the release of the same 'feel good' brain chemicals, e.g., dopamine and endorphins, as do opioids – and the opioid-specific placebo effect.*

I, bias aside, recommend exploring *'Brain Mediation'* – a very pure and potent form of meditation that can be done, in quick bursts, right throughout the day in background mode, i.e., while doing mundane tasks like brushing your teeth, taking a shower, or sitting in a waiting room for a doctor's appointment. The notion of *'befriending the brain'* is key to *'Brain Mediation'*. It is about thinking and treating your brain as your best friend. You start each day, first thing, by wishing your brain a *'good morning'*. Given the pain-brain connection, and the undeniable potential of mind over matter, there can only be an upside to such a relationship.

It is all happening 'up there' in your head, and the more *sway* you can have with your brain the better.

Yoga, though it can be physically more demanding, is another oft recommended, and often highly successful, option. In reality *any exercise* is likely to be better than nothing because exercise too will trigger the release of some of the brain's 'feel good' chemicals.

Never lose sight of the 'check engine' light analogy. Whenever evaluating a supposed CPS-related treatment option try and determine whether it really is trying to replace <u>THE light</u> or whether it, yet again, is trying, pointlessly, to replace the brake pads or the catalytic converter probe.

Please take the time to think about what you have read and gleamed from this chapter. It could really help you. Do not dismiss, downplay or choose to ignore this vital pain-brain connection. It is so important when it comes to understanding CPS, not to mention dealing with and coping with CPS. CPS sucks. Nobody is going to deny that. You have to learn to somehow live with CPS on a daily basis. And appreciating the pain-brain linkage will help you in this difficult, but necessary, quest.

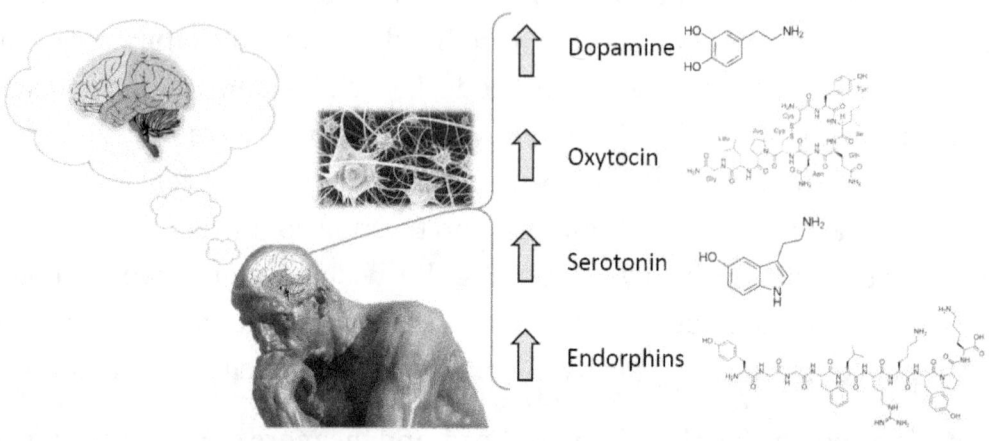

Brain's chief *'feel good'* chemicals

Some of the chemistry behind 'Brain Meditation',
though it is also true that similar results may
also be possible with other forms of meditation.

NDC 0603-1880-16

LIDOCAINE PATCH 5%

R$_X$ only

Each adhesive patch contains:
Lidocaine 700 mg (50 mg per gram adhesive) in an aqueous base.
Methylparaben and propylparaben as preservatives.

30 PATCHES
30 Envelopes
Containing 1 Patch Each

Usual Dosage: Apply up to 3 patches. See package insert for
complete prescribing information.

Store at 25°C (77°F); excursions permitted to 15°-30°C (59°-86°F).

WARNING: Keep used and unused patches out of the reach of
children, pets and others.

TAKEAWAYS:
CHAPTER 4 – PAIN & THE BRAIN

ൠ *All pain is in the brain* **irrespective** of Central Pain Syndrome (CPS) – since all perceptions of pain, in all humans, occur in the brain.

ൠ Three things that are different when you have CPS: **1)** brain, unintentionally, *amplifies **all*** of its pain responses (so-called *hyperalgesia*), **2)** brain receives *confusing/false* pain signals, and **3)** emotional distress, already *heighted* by the pain, causes pain to be *further amplified*.

ൠ The 'Check Engine' light analogy: *the pain* of CPS is the faulty, malfunctioning <u>light</u> (due to a disorder of the central nervous system) and <u>nothing else</u> – as such you can try to fix everything else within the car, but the light will stay on because the <u>*fault is in the light*</u> and not what it is supposed to be signaling.

ൠ The joint or muscle pain of CPS, *as with fibromyalgia*, is not due to actual inflammation, injury or infection – as such, trying to seek treatment for a non-existent inflammation, injury or infection is not going to help relieve the pain.

ൠ Anesthetics, such as lidocaine, work by blocking nerves from being able to transmit pain signals to the CNS, while opioids set out to reduce the perception of pain by triggering the release of brain chemicals.

ൠ Hyperalgesia is the bane of CPS, and in what is indeed a cruel twist, prolonged use of opioids can make hyperalgesia worse!

ൠ The possibilities of *mind over matter* should never be underestimated; *meditation*, particularly 'Brain Meditation', an easy way to try and gain some ongoing benefits – with *yoga*, albeit physically more demanding, yet another option.

ൠ Continually try to exploit the placebo effect by always trying to be *really, really hyped* as to how well a new drug or a treatment option is going to work.

5.
DIAGNOSIS

There is **no** chemical test, _as yet_, for diagnosing Central Pain Syndrome.

There is, as such, no blood tests, spinal fluid analysis (via a lumbar puncture), urine test, or 'culture' that can indicate the presence of CPS.

Blood tests, lumbar punctures and other tests, however, may still be used to detect possible causes for CPS hitherto undiagnosed (e.g., meningitis or late stage Lyme disease). In some cases further tests may be done to eliminate additional conditions (such as, diabetic pain, early stage MS, neurological complications of chronic herpes or Lupus). In all cases these tests are for finding or excluding possible causes – rather than to confirm or deny the presence of CPS. This is important to keep in mind.

CPS, therefore, has to be diagnosed based on the symptoms and the patient's medical history relative to the long list of possible causes of CPS.

CT or **MRI** scans will _invariably_ be used, early on, to try and detect any obvious damage to the central nervous system – particularly to the neck or spinal column. When available MRIs tend to be preferred, though even X-rays may sometimes suffice.

Imaging, with its ever-increasing sophistication, could uncover, previously unsuspected, tumors, injuries, hemorrhages, aneurysms and other damage. That is never good news, but at least it would explain the onset of CPS.

If you *think* you have CPS it will not be a bad idea, if you can, to get some good imaging done of your spinal column, neck and brain. It is not unusual to be told of various damage that you may not have been aware.

Following a neck X-ray (a longtime ago) I was asked *'when where you in a car accident?'* Since I had not been in any major vehicular accident, that I could recall, I was bemused. I was told I had neck vertebrae damage most often associated with serious whiplash. To this day I have no idea as to how I damaged those vertebrae. But, you can see, clear as day, on the X-ray, that all is not right. I have no idea how this could have happened.

So, there could be clues unbeknownst to you as to a possible cause for the CPS that are hard to overlook on the medical imaging.

If you have a medical history that involves the central nervous system, spinal column or anything related to them (e.g., brain injury, spinal surgery or herniated discs), doctors are unlikely to look any further – provided, of course, that other 'biggies' have been discounted.

CPS following spinal surgery is fairly common. It is strange that patients are not routinely appraised of this possibility beforehand or at least during the recovery phase. As such it comes as a very unpleasant surprise.

If a cause for the symptoms of CPS remains underlined elusive, sufferers will, nonetheless, get *treated for the symptoms*. This, of course, makes a lot of sense and is increasingly becoming *the norm*.

There are no CPS-specific drugs or treatment regimens. Treatment options for CPS are, thus, invariably aimed at trying to reduce the severity of the symptoms – in most cases the pain, the burning sensations and the emotional distress.

Consequently, it does not really matter whether there is, or is not, a definitive diagnosis of CPS.

There is technology that can detect minute changes in electrical activity within the nervous system, in particular the CNS. This technology is referred to as '*Evoked Potentials*' – where the 'potentials' denote the change in electrical 'voltages', while 'evoked' signifies that these electrical changes are realized using external stimulation. In this context, lasers can be used to evoke pain responses.

So, there is a *'Laser Evoked Potential'* (LEP) test that can be used to determine pain-related *nerve damage* in or around the CNS. This testing is typically considered to be 'extravagant' and 'unnecessary' in the case of CPS. Trying to obtain possible confirmation of nerve damage does not help in identifying a cause or influence the treatment. The symptoms of CPS are proof enough, most of the time, that there is underlying nerve damage somewhere in the body.

A RELUCTANCE TO DIAGNOSE CPS?

There appears to be, at least in the U.S., a hesitancy among doctors when it comes to telling a patient that they have or might have CPS.

Even when a doctor suspects CPS that diagnosis may not be volunteered unless specifically asked about it.

Quite often a doctor may settle for a diagnosis of fibromyalgia and leave it at that without mentioning CPS.

There could be multiple reasons for this disinclination:

1. Lack of *determinicity*: the lack of any tests (at present) that conclusively identify CPS means any diagnosis will always appear to be an opinion.

    With fibromyalgia, there is, at least, the 9 pairs of *tender points* that can be checked and reported upon. Though the effectiveness of this tender point test is now questioned, it has remained an accepted basis for diagnosis. Thus, a doctor finding pain in at least 11 of the possible 18 tender points can say, categorically, that you have fibromyalgia. So, the fibromyalgia diagnosis appears to be very scientific and conclusive – even if that is not entirely the case!

2. Does not influence treatment: given there are **no** CPS-specific treatment options, a diagnosis of CPS does not make any real difference as to the treatment regimen specified to a patient.

3. CPS is hard to *explain*, *justify* and *rationalize*: unless they already had some familiarity with CPS, a patient on first being told they have CPS will, understandably, have lots of questions, concerns, uncertainty and anxiety. And, as you probably have already seen, there aren't that many specific answers a doctor can provide to explain the '*why*' and '*what*' of CPS. You just end up going round-and-round the CNS disorder explanation. Plus, there are no specific assurances that can be made. So, given that it does not in any way influence the treatment options, it is much 'easier' not to mention CPS and just talk about the symptoms and what can be done to reduce their severity.

4. The *phantom nature*: though this is also true for fibromyalgia, CPS can come across as being *psychosomatic*, i.e., without an identifiable physical basis. While the pain is very real, what is actually causing it remains hard to explain. This is particularly so in the case of joint and muscle pain if there is no actual inflammation, infection or injury. Thus, as in #3 (↑), it is often just easier to treat the symptoms and leave a possible diagnosis of CPS unsaid.

5. Insurance and reimbursement factors: probably more of an issue in the U.S. than in other countries, but there could be instances when it is easier to appease 'bureaucracy', particularly so when there is money at stake, with a diagnosis other than that of CPS.

The bottom line here is that there is a possibility, especially in the U.S., that you might not be diagnosed as having CPS – even if you do and your doctor knows that you do! But, it will *not affect* the treatment you will receive.

That you have not been diagnosed with CPS does not mean, for sure, that you do not have CPS. It could just mean that you might have CPS, but your doctor is unwilling to tell you as such. Maybe you have been told you have fibromyalgia or just unspecified, generalized, chronic pain. The latter could be always be a valid diagnosis – independent of CPS.

A claim made by some that CPS is not readily diagnosed because doctors are not familiar with it is hard to rationalize. While it is possible a general practitioner may not be that familiar with CPS, it is hard to believe a doctor specializing in pain would not know about CPS. The notion of 'central pain' is hard to overlook if you deal in pain.

That said, it is also true that CPS is not well understood across both the medical and scientific communities. Statements to that effect can be readily found online. It is a fact that not much research has been done, to-date, on CPS. But, that is beginning to change as you will see below – in terms of the 'future of CPS'.

If you believe you have CPS and want it confirmed, you may have to confront your doctor. You may have to specifically ask: "*do I have Central Pain Syndrome?*" However, in the end, we end up back to the same conclusion. It does not matter whether you are diagnosed with CPS or not, if you have the symptoms of CPS you will get treated for those symptoms irrespective of what the paperwork claims is your condition.

THE HISTORY & FUTURE OF CPS

Central Pain Syndrome is not a newly discovered condition. It has been known for over 100 years.

The first specific description of CPS can be dated back to **1891**. This was when Ludwig Edinger, a German neurologist and the co-founder of the University of Frankfurt, attributed it to being related to a damaged thalamus in the brain – most likely due to a stroke. (Refer to '*Stroke Related*' in chapter 3.)

Fifteen years later two French neurologists, Joseph Jules Dejerine and Gustave Roussy, published a paper on *'Thalamic Syndrome'* where they described *post-stroke pain* and associated that pain with the *thalamic region* of the brain. This pain came to be known as: *thalamic (pain) syndrome* or *Dejerine–Roussy syndrome*.

For the next sixty-years, or more, 'central pain' was always thought of in the context of thalamic pain syndrome.

But that started to change when doctors and researchers realized this pain was not just limited to those that had suffered a stroke. That was when the notion of CPS, associated with any damage or injury to the central nervous system, came to be. The *'central'* in the name points to the association with the **central** *nervous system*.

By the 1990s 'central pain' had gained considerable traction. However, it has not received the research attention it deserves in its *own right*, though over the last decade there has been considerable funding for research related to brain disorders, neurosciences and mental health. Cancer, diabetes, heart disease, Alzheimer's, HIV/AIDS and even obesity invariably get more attention due to their higher profile in society and the media. Hence, the oft heard claim that CPS is not that well understood (at present). But that, as you will shortly see, is luckily beginning to change.

Multiple sclerosis, given that the nerve damage could be seen with a microscope, was identified as a specific disease in 1868 (i.e., twenty years ahead of CPS). However, it was well into the next century before the exact nature of MS was finally understood, with the first effective treatments only becoming available in the 1990s.

While chronic, inexplicable, widespread pain is not anything new to the medical community, the term 'fibromyalgia' itself only first came to be in the 1970s. Prior to that a variety of names such as *'muscular rheumatism'*, *'fibrositis'*, *'psychogenic rheumatism'*, and *'neurasthenia'* had been used to describe such pain – with *'psychogenic'* suggesting that its cause might be psychological rather than physical.

The diagnosis based on the *nine-pairs of tender points* was introduced by the 'American College of Rheumatology' (ACR) in 1990. It, at least among doctors genuinely specializing in pain, no longer carries the weight it once did. As mentioned in chapter 1 there is escalating controversy surrounding fibromyalgia, with some doctors questioning the validity of the diagnosis while others are questioning whether it is more psychological than physical. But, as with CPS, there could be some light emerging at the end of the tunnel as the study of overall pain enters a new phase.

CPS in the Future

Over the last few years **Central Sensitization (Syndrome)** has been gaining considerable attention and research funding (as was originally mentioned in chapter 1).

'*Chronic pain*' in the U.S. is now being openly described as an <u>epidemic</u>. A 2016 study by U.S. National Institute of Health (NIH) indicated that around **50 million** Americans suffer from either chronic or severe pain (CPS sufferers, of course, among these). That is a BIG number that cannot be ignored – in that it represents 16% of the population. It is larger, by far, than those in the U.S. with diabetes, cancer or heart disease!

Chronic pain impacts industry and commerce. Absenteeism and loss of productivity is one issue, whereas the growing number of folks genuinely seeking disability status due to their constant pain is another. Treating pain is now placing a huge, and ever ballooning, financial burden on health care systems, the insurance industry and social services organizations.

Moreover, the highly destructive and costly *opioid use epidemic* is directly tied to the vast number of people struggling with chronic pain. Consequently, there is now significant interest, motivation and incentive to try and get a good handle on chronic pain -- governments and corporations eager to provide funding. Much of the new research on this front is being done under the umbrella of *Central Sensitization*.

Central Sensitization is a broader categorization than just CPS or fibromyalgia. It is described as the *nervous system condition* that is responsible for causing and maintaining chronic pain – *in all of its* various guises.

Hyperalgesia is one of two key components that make up central sensitization. The other has to do with a patient experiencing noticeable pain as a result of interactions that should not be painful – e.g., being lightly touched, the feel of clothing/bedding or a gentle breeze. Yes, as with hyperalgesia, this too is a known characteristic of CPS. The medical term for it is *allodynia* – Greek for 'other pain'.

Central Sensitization = Hyperalgesia + Allodynia.

Any and all advances made in terms of central sensitization (syndrome) will have a bearing on CPS. Therefore, going forward look for news and developments on CS rather than just CPS and/or fibromyalgia. It is even possible that a prior diagnosis of CPS may get amended to CS – as CS becomes the 'big umbrella' that covers nearly everything to do with chronic pain.

The bottom line here is that the future holds promise. Chronic pain is finally getting the attention it should have received a longtime ago. There may not be any miracle cures in the short-term, but at least, with CS, many cogs have finally been engaged in the hope of achieving such a goal – if that is at all feasible.

TAKEAWAYS:
CHAPTER 5 – DIAGNOSIS

ෆ There is, *as yet*, **no** blood test, spinal fluid analysis, urine test or 'culture' that can be used to diagnose Central Pain Syndrome – but, these, and more, may be used to detect possible CPS causes previously undiagnosed or to eliminate other conditions.

ෆ CPS invariably has to be diagnosed based on the symptoms and the patient's medical history – especially as it relates to anything to do with the central nervous system.

ෆ Medical imaging, in particular MRIs, will often be used to confirm or detect additional injury/damage to the central nervous system.

ෆ It is increasingly the case that doctors will *treat the symptoms*, irrespective of a diagnosis of CPS given that there is no specific treatment options unique to CPS.

ෆ It may not be that unusual to find doctors, even specialist pain doctors, for various reasons, to be somewhat reluctant to openly diagnose CPS – and may opt to say it is fibromyalgia instead.

ෆ While it is true CPS is still ill-understood, the assertion that doctors are unfamiliar with it is probably unwarranted, particularly in the case of qualified pain doctors.

ෆ If you suspect you have CPS it may be best to address it directly with your doctor rather than waiting for the doctor to bring it up; i.e., don't wait to be told, ask your doctor whether you have Central Pain Syndrome.

ෆ Central pain related research and study is now increasingly falling under the *Central Sensitization (Syndrome)* umbrella – which is 'OK' from a CPS perspective since the key pain-related factors of CPS fall squarely within what is covered by CSS.

6.
TREATMENT

There is both good and bad news when it comes to the treatment of Central Pain Syndrome.

On the good news front it has to be said that it *may be possible* to find a treatment options that will somehow *reduce* the pain/discomfort of CPS for *some period of time* each day. Some, *with luck*, may even be able to gain considerable relief, or indeed be nearly pain-free, for longer stretches of time. It is also the case that new treatment options continue to become available – the affordable, wireless TENS units, from the likes of '*Aleve*' and '*Icy Hot*', but a recent example.

The development of a completely new type of pain relief medication is nearing completion. It is an opioid, but one that sets out, from the get-go, to be as close to the body's own natural, pain relieving opioids, e.g., *endorphins*. The expectation being that these new drugs will offer considerable levels of pain management without the adverse side effects of today's pain medications, particularly the opioids. However, given the long-drawn-out evaluations and clinical trials required these drugs are unlikely to be approved for widespread use, at least in the U.S., till sometime beyond 2021.

There are also some 'experimental' (or 'investigational') treatment options that have proved to be successful on occasion. In addition, finding viable cures for chronic pain has now become a major priority for many in the medical, scientific and pharmaceutical circles (as mentioned at the end of the last chapter) – with the unignorable *opioid use epidemic*, that has touched so many lives, a major driving force. So, there is definite *hope* that increasingly more effective cures for CPS (and chronic pain) will be forthcoming.

So, the good news is: *'encouraging to an extent and with promise in the future'*.

The bad news is that there is **no cure**, *as yet*, for CPS. Furthermore, finding an effective treatment to deal with the woes of CPS can be difficult, *'hit-or-miss'*, capricious, and as such, extremely *frustrating for all*. To make matters worse, it is not unusual for *treatment tolerance* to set-in (often quite quickly), necessitating frequent changes to dosages or the entire treatment regime. And then, when it comes to the drugs (some of which have to be *'heavy-duty'* in order to succeed), there are the inevitable *side-effects*, many not *'so pleasant'* - to put it mildly!

To compound matters further, when it comes to CPS, there is no consistency in the effectiveness of a treatment across patients. ***What might work for one patient will not work for another***. So, treatments have to be patient-specific and determined through an exasperating process of *'trial-and-error'*. As such, doctors and patients are more than happy to go with *'whatever that works'* – even if it makes no medical sense. This also sometimes means that doctors and patients will turn a blind eye towards potential *consequences down-the-road*. The emphasis always being on what will work *right now*, as opposed to giving any thought to the future.

Whatever caused the CPS, if it is known (e.g., epilepsy), will continue to be treated – if possible and feasible.

In the case of CPS attributed to prior *neck or spinal column problems*, there will, understandably, be a dogged determination to keep on trying to reduce any pain **that may be** originating from the original site.

And then, overnight, what might have been working quite well will cease to work, and you are back to the drawing board yet again!

That is CPS.

It is fairly routine to rely on a combination of drugs and/or treatment options (e.g., use of multiple drugs, lidocaine patches and a TENS unit). But, suddenly, the pain levels that had been maintained at relatively manageable rates could shoot off the charts. Now, you have to work out which drug or drugs needs to be reevaluated, replaced or increased.

Yes, the stress of it all adds to the problems of CPS. Another vicious circle when it comes to CPS.

So, in the case of treatment options, CPS sufferers invariably are forced to deal with hard choices, imperfect compromises, constant uncertainty and the knowledge that *'things will not improve anytime soon'*.

In many instances, despite treatment, there will always be some level of pain, discomfort and emotional distress. That is CPS.

The treatment options for CPS fall into two categories: **standard therapy regimens** and **experimental/investigational therapy regimens**. The latter, which involves brain stimulation and/or neurosurgery is usually a last resort when most other treatment options have been exhausted.

STANDARD THERAPY REGIMEN

Standard therapy for CPS will include one or more of the treatment options listed below. Typically, *multiple options* will be employed in parallel, with multiple drug combinations.

1. Medications taken orally in the form of **pills, tablets or capsules**. This continues to be the primary and preferred means of trying to contain the symptoms of CPS – and, more often than not, the first resort in the battle against CPS. *The oral medication options for CPS are discussed in more detail **below**,* in the next section.

2. Medication delivered **through the skin** (i.e., *transdermal*), in particular local anesthetics such as ***Lidocaine*** delivered via 'long-

acting' (i.e., 10+ hours) patches (as mentioned in chapter 4). Cream and spray variants may also be prescribed though their effects may not be as long-lasting as that of a patch. [Good patches, given their effectiveness, can be *expensive*, e.g., $24 per patch, in the U.S.]

3. **Injections**, typically of the type used for back pain relief, and as such including:

   a. **Epidural steroid injections** - a combination of *local anesthetic* (e.g., Lidocaine) and *steroids* injected close to the *spinal column*. Synthetic *corticosteroids* (*corticoids*) which can help reduce inflammation are what is most used in terms of steroids.

   b. **Selective nerve root block (SNRB)** – though often used as a diagnostic to determine which *spinal nerves* (branching out of the spinal column) may be causing pain, it can also be used as a means of temporarily reducing pain caused by a pinched or inflamed spinal nerve. 'Live X-ray' (called 'fluoroscopy') is employed to help guide the needle towards the target nerve. The injection may contain a *local anesthetic* (typically Lidocaine), a *corticosteroid* or a combination of both. What differentiates this from an '*epidural*' (above) is that it is targeted at a specific spinal nerve – hence the '*selective*' in the name.

   c. **Facet joint block** – facet joints are on the backside of the spinal column; on the other side from the spinal discs. They are what enables the spine to be flexible so that you can bend and twist. A facet joint block is an injection of *local anesthetic*, 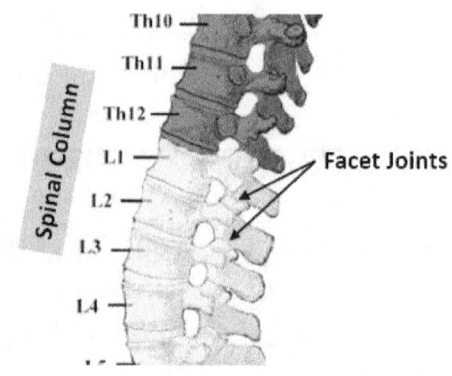 *corticosteroid*s or both, to one or more of the joints to numb pain.

d. **Sacroiliac joint block** – the sacroiliac joints or SI joints (SIJ), as shown in the diagram below, are in the pelvis; one on each side. Damage or inflammation to one or both of the SI joints can result in lower back pain. The 'joint block' is an *anesthetic/corticosteroid* injection (similar to those mentioned above) delivered close to the SI joint.

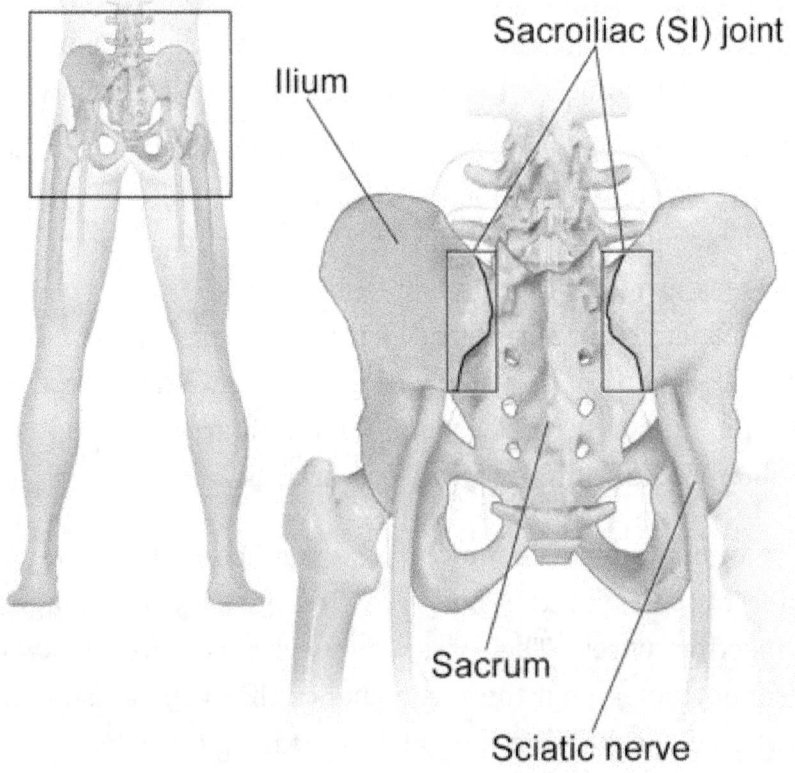

Sacroiliac Joints

-- from Wikipedia

4. **Rhizotomy** – is a relatively minor *surgical procedure*, done with *needles*, that attempts to block pain by trying to selectively *destroy* (i.e., deaden), problem-causing spinal nerves. The nerves are destroyed using *heat* – the required heat generated by sending high frequency electrical 'impulses' through a metal needle. As with a 'selective nerve root block' (above) 'live X-ray' (i.e., 'fluoroscopy') is

used to make sure the needle is in the right place. Rhizotomy is most often used on *facet joints* (above).

5. **Electrical Nerve Simulation: External & _Internal_** – is the therapeutic treatment of muscle pain/spasms via (gentle) electrical stimulation of nerves. The stimulation, in the form of electrical pulses, attempts to reduce pain in two ways: **1/** by trying to *block pain signals* from reaching the central nervous system, and **2/** by trying to coax the brain into producing more *endorphins*, the body's own natural painkiller (described in chapter 4 and below).

If this is done through the skin it is called **TENS** – *transcutaneous electrical nerve stimulation*, where '*cutaneous*' refers to it being skin-based. Machines that perform TENS, via adhesive patches affixed to the areas needing attention, are called TENS units. TENS units are now available in wired and wireless forms. 'Heavy duty' ones typically require a prescription, though the latest, wireless consumer units (priced at around U.S. $50) are said to be as effective as older, prescription-only, wired variants.

Wired units support four or more patches that can be placed on different parts of the body, limited just by the length of the connecting wires. The wires, however, can be 'awkward' and uncomfortable – and there is a chance that you can sometimes get unwanted shocks from the patches wearing thin, the gel applied to the patches (for better conductivity) being uneven or a gap in the insulation of the metal connectors on the patches. The wireless options typically can only support two patches since the small, battery-powered 'impulse unit' has to be directly attached to the back of the patches. Some units come with a remote control to adjust the intensity and 'pattern' of the impulses. The wireless units thus cover less area, though in theory it would be possible to use multiple units at the same time on different parts of the body.

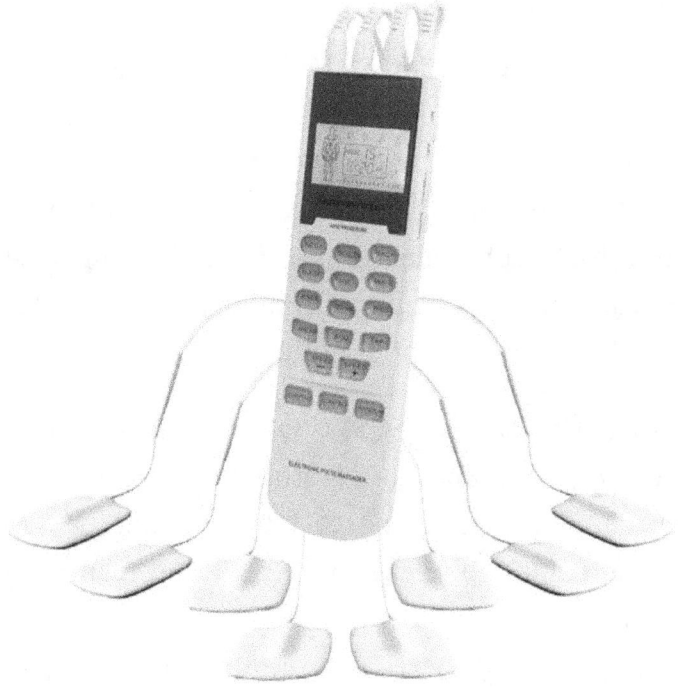

A wired, FDA-approved TENS unit, the '*HealthmateForever YK15AB*', available at Amazon.com for under U.S. $30.

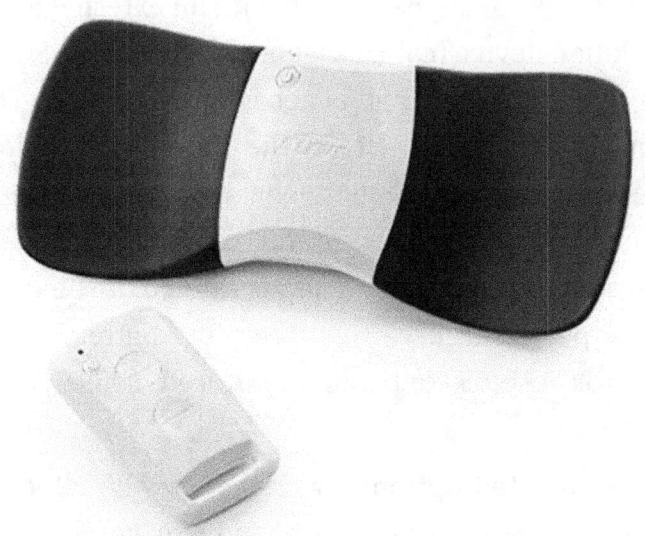

The '*Aleve Direct Therapy*' wireless TENS unit,
with remote control, that holds *two patches*
on the backside of the unit, and now
available in stores and online for under U.S. $40.

Internal, implanted options

Peripheral Nerve Stimulation (PNS) is a procedure, performed on an out-patient basis with local anesthetic, where thin electrodes are inserted into the body – along the path of peripheral nerves. The electrodes can be connected to an external unit or to a small, battery-powered, remote controlled unit, that is also *implanted under the skin*. It is customary to begin with a trial period using an external unit before the fully implanted option is undertaken.

Spinal Cord Stimulation (SCS) is when the electrical stimulation is done directly to the spinal cord (rather than to the nerves branching out from it). The goal being to try and stop pain signals from reaching the central nervous system by intercepting them at the 'boundary'.

As with PNS it is typical to evaluate the effectiveness of this approach using an external unit – connected to inserted 'wires' placed against the spinal cord (using local anesthetic).

The implanted option is usually only undertaken if a patient reports a 50% to 70% decrease in pain with an external unit. The implanted stimulation device (called a 'generator') used in SCS tends to require more major surgery than is necessary with PNS. The unit is placed, under general anesthetic, in the buttock or abdomen – with the surgery typically lasting between an hour to two hours. The battery inside the implanted generator can be charged via an external, cordless recharger. The battery is rated to last between 7 to 9 years; with repeat surgery required for battery replacement. The generator is operated and monitored using a handheld remote controller.

These implanted options can *sometimes* be effective – though, yet again, they are not a cure *per se* and *may not work* in all instances.

At some point during the treatment of CPS a pain doctor is likely to bring up these in-body stimulation possibilities. They should be contemplated without considerable deliberation and consultation. Costs and insurance coverage can further complicate matters.

6. **Psychiatric care, psychotherapy** and **counselling** to address the psychological aspect of CPS, knowing that depression and anxiety, so often the inescapable *side-effect* of CPS, are also *contributing factors* that worsen *hyperalgesia*.

7. **Physical therapy** and exercise.

8. **Meditation** and **yoga** for reducing stress and calming the mind.

9. **Medical marijuana**.

10. **Alternate therapies**, such as *acupuncture*, along the '*whatever might work*' premise, with the recognition that the placebo effect, as described in chapter 4, is not to be underestimated.

ORAL MEDICATIONS

Given their ease of administration, a wide variety of oral medications, in numerous combinations, are invariably used in the treatment of CPS. They are always meant to reduce/contain the symptoms, in particular the pain, *rather than to be cures*. The types of oral medications used include:

a. **Traditional painkillers** (i.e., *analgesic drugs*):

In particular *acetaminophen* (a.k.a. paracetamol) (e.g., **Tylenol** & Panadol) or *nonsteroidal anti-inflammatory drugs* (**NSAIDs**) such as *ibuprofen* (e.g., **Advil** & **Motrin**).

The effectiveness of these traditional painkillers when it comes to CPS is questioned and *controversial*. Many maintain that they provide little or no relief. Nonetheless, doctors will often suggest one or more of such painkillers, sometimes in tandem (e.g., Tylenol & Advil together) – albeit, sometimes as a '*take as needed*' adjunct to other treatment options, including additional oral medications.

There are, of course (and alas), side effects to all of these drugs, some of them serious. Acetaminophen is linked to acute liver failure. Thus, it is **not** always advisable to believe that all the so called 'traditional painkillers' are unlikely to have any adverse consequences -- especially if taken in high doses. Note, that acetaminophen can sometimes be found in cough and cold medication, not to mention opioid combinations (e.g., Vicodin, Percocet & Xodol). As such, you could end up taking more than you had realized or intended.

b. **Opioids** & **Opioid/Analgesic combinations**:

The use of opioids for the treatment of CPS is <u>controversial</u>, troubling and divisive.

Many in the medical and scientific communities claim, categorically, that opioids are not effective, in general, when it comes to CPS – with some even going onto say they should ***not*** be prescribed to most CPS sufferers. There are, however, CPS sufferers and doctors that will vehemently *disagree*. Opioid-based treatment definitely falls into the '*whatever that seems to work, never mind the logic or consequences*' approach to the treatment of CPS. There are plenty of doctors that will subscribe to this because it makes the patient happy and '*it is good for business*'.

Some CPS sufferers, especially those with neck or back issues, may have been taking opioids prior to the onset of CPS. They may opt to continue with opioids, irrespective. Giving up opioids can be hard, very hard – and that is putting it mildly.

Opioids, initially in the form of *opium* from the '*opium poppy seed*', have been used for many centuries as an extremely effective foil against pain. *Morphine*, first 'extracted' from opium poppies in the early 1800s, probably is the best-known example. The term '*opioid*', introduced in the 1950s, indicates this connection with opium.

Opioid = opium + '*oid*', meaning '*opium like*'.

The human body naturally produces its own opioids! These are our body's internal pain-relieving chemicals. They are called ***endogenous opioids*** or *endogenous peptides* (where 'peptides' is a technical name for short chains of amino acids). *'Endogenous'* basically meaning *'naturally occurring'* (and in this case, within our bodies).

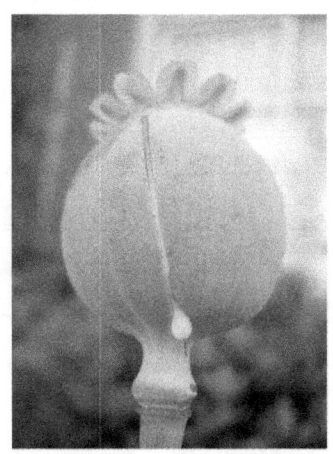

Opium poppy
seed pod.

Endorphins, produced by the central nervous system and the pituitary gland (at the base of the brain), are one of these *endogenous opioids*. Endorphins <u>suppress the transmission of pain signals</u> to the brain – thereby reducing pain sensations (per the discussion in chapter 4). Endorphins may also be responsible for making one feel *euphoric* – given that opioids are known for this.

Other *endogenous opioids* produced naturally within the body include: *dynorphins*, *enkephalins* and *endomorphins*. [That last name actually meaning *'morphine naturally produced within the body'*.] All these *endogenous opioids*, in one way or another, influence how the body reacts to pain, arousal, sedation, etc.

Opioid medications work by supplementing (and in some cases overwhelming) the *endogenous opioids*.

This supplementation, particularly over time, interferes with the brain's chemical production and chemical balance – the production of *dopamine*, the body's 'feel good' chemical, being just one of the casualties. It is this disruption of brain chemistry that causes all the issues associated with opioids.

Opioid medication, not counting the opioid/analgesic combinations, comes in three different classes based on how they are produced.

The table below characterizes these three classes of opioids and lists *some* examples.

OPIOID MEDICATION		
Narcotic – i.e., pain reducing drugs		
Opiates		
NATURAL	**SEMI-SYNTHETIC**	**SYNTHETIC**
Directly from the opium poppy	Contains material from the opium poppy	All artificial
Examples: • Codeine • Morphine	• Hydrocodone • Oxycodone *(OxyContin)* • *Heroin* • Hydromorphone • Oxymorphone • Buprenorphine	• Levorphanol *(5 times stronger than morphine)* • Meperidine • Fentanyl • Methadone • Tapentadol *(Nucynta, Palexia)* • Tramadol

More often than not opioids, especially in the U.S., are prescribed in opioid/acetaminophen or opioid/NSAID (e.g., ibuprofen) combinations. Such combinations are said to be longer acting, but it appears that the primary rationale for combining the drugs into a single pill is to avoid the availability of pure opioids on their own. *Some* of the more popular of these combinations are as follows:

Hydrocodone/Acetaminophen: Vicodin, Xodol, Lorcet, Norco, Lortab, Hycet, etc.

Oxycodone/Acetaminophen: Percocet, Endocet, Roxicet, etc.

Codeine/Acetaminophen: Tylenol with Codeine, etc.

Tramadol/Acetaminophen: Ultracet, Ultram; Tramal, etc.

[Acetaminophen (i.e., Tylenol), as mentioned above, can cause serious liver damage. Therefore, care should be taken to monitor total dosage taking into account the amount included in hybrid drugs such as these.]

Hydrocodone/Ibuprofen: Xylon, Ibudone, Reprexain, etc.

Oxycodone/ Ibuprofen: Percodan, etc.

In the U.S., in particular, there is increasing pressure on doctors, in the form of guidelines and prescription monitoring, to be extra diligent when it comes to opioids.

A study from 2013, available on the U.S. government sponsored 'National Center for Biotechnology Information' (NCBI), titled <u>'Opioids for neuropathic pain'</u> states: *'The use of opioids for neuropathic pain remains controversial'* as well as *'Analgesic efficacy of opioids in chronic neuropathic pain is subject to considerable uncertainty'*. Given that CPS is indeed a neuropathic condition these observations are applicable and relevant.

The 'National Organization for Rare Disorders' (NORD) is a U.S.-based non-profit dedicated to patient advocacy. CPS is a condition covered by NORD. Its discussion of CPS includes this statement: *'Opioids such as morphine or levorphanol are not effective in the vast majority of cases and are actually contraindicated for most patients'*.

In the context of CPS, opioids are known to make hyperalgesia more acute and worsen depression and anxiety. This further *exaggerates* the pain amplification ↔ emotional distress *vicious cycle* described in chapter 4. The *'contraindication'* mentioned in the NORD statement above has much to do with this. This phenomenon is known by terms such as: *opioid-induced hyperalgesia, opioid-induced abnormal pain sensitivity* and *paradoxical hyperalgesia.* Suffice to say that, as with so much to do with opioids, there is considerable controversy as to whether *opioid-induced hyperalgesia* is real.

But, there are CPS patients who will claim, quite passionately, that opioids, even with very long-term use, continue to provide them with some level of noticeable relief – and that opioids are one of the few things *'that works'*.

Nothing can be generalized when it comes to CPS (other than, alas, the fact that, opioids or no opioids, there is no known cure, as yet, for CPS).

c. **Antiepileptic** & **Antidepressant** medication:

There is considerable evidence and agreement (from all sides) that certain *antiepileptic/anticonvulsant* and *antidepressant* medications can be rather effective in treating CPS – though they should not be looked at as permanent cures (since that is unlikely to be the case).

Pregabalin, best known by its brand name *Lyrica,* is a good example. Pregabalin was synthesized in 1990 as an anticonvulsant. But, following U.S. FDA approval in 2004, it has been very successfully marketed by Pfizer, in the form of Lyrica, to also treat *fibromyalgia, (diabetic) neuropathic pain* and *generalized anxiety.* Given this relevance, in particular to fibromyalgia, it is often prescribed to CPS patients – usually as the first line of defense against the pain.

Duloxetine, marketed as *Cymbalta* by Eli Lilly, is another example. It was developed in the mid-1980s as a treatment for major depressive disorder and generalized anxiety disorder. It too got FDA approval in 2004, for treating both *depression* and *diabetic neuropathic pain.* Since then fibromyalgia and neuropathic pain, independent of diabetes, has been added to the list.

All these drugs, of course, work by '*blocking-and-tackling*' various brain chemicals and thereby altering, temporarily be it, brain chemistry. And given that we now know that pain is '*in the brain*', you can appreciate how modifying the chemistry could affect the way the brain handles pain.

These drugs work differently to opioids – hence why they are not classed as such or called pain relievers. Nonetheless, these drugs too have side effects and consequences – in some cases relatively severe; e.g., increase in suicidal tendencies. These drugs are typically only available via prescription. So, there will be some degree of medical oversight. That is good. Always keep in mind that these drugs are powerful and that they are 'altering' the basic chemistry of *your brain*. **They can well and truly mess with your brain!**

Some of the drugs, from these two categories, that are used to treat CPS include:

Antiepileptic drugs (AEDs) & Anticonvulsants: *Gabapentin* (Neurontin), *Pregabalin* (Lyrica), *Carbamazepine* (Tegretol), *Topiramate* (Topamax) and *Lamotrigine* (Lamictal).

Midazolam (Versed), though primarily an anesthetic and sedative, is also sometimes used to treat seizures. It, usually in injection-form, has had some success in reliving the symptoms of CPS.

Antidepressants: *Amitriptyline* (Elavil) and *Duloxetine* (Cymbalta).

Ketamine (brand name 'Ketalar', street name 'Special K') is a powerful, 'disorienting' and hallucinogenic synthesized anesthetic widely used by veterinarians to sedate large animals. It is used in some instances to control chronic and post-operative pain. It is not a pain medication typically prescribed for CPS. Of late it is being *evaluated* as a highly effective and quick acting antidepressant. U.S. FDA, however, has yet to approve it for use as such.

d. **Muscle relaxants:**

Muscle relaxants act as sedatives for the central nervous system. Hence, the applicability when it comes to CPS. A muscle relaxant will typically be used in conjunction with other drugs and treatment. It is unlikely that a muscle relaxant on its own will be adequate to deal effectively with the pain of CPS.

Examples of *some* of the muscle relaxants that may be used with CPS include: *Methocarbamol* (Robaxin), *Cyclobenzaprine* (Flexeril, Amrix), *Chlorzoxazone* (Lorzone), *Baclofen* (Lioresal) and *Tizanidine* (Zanaflex).

e. **Antiarrhythmic agents:**

These are drugs used to treat irregular heart rhythms – hence the '*rhythmic*' in the name. At least one of them, i.e., *Mexiletine* (Mexitil), is said to be effective in the treatment of CPS – though it is not approved or recommended for use when it comes to neuropathic pain. So, if prescribed, it will be '*off label*' – so to speak.

Interestingly, *lidocaine* (talked about earlier as a local anesthetic), in injection form (i.e., intravenously), serves as a very useful antiarrhythmic agent.

f. **Sedatives, Anti-Anxiety Medications** (e.g., *Benzodiazepines* such as Xanax, Klonopin, Ativan, Valium, etc.) & **Sleep Aids.**

EXPERIMENTAL/INVESTIGATION THERAPIES

These are '*last resort*', '*extreme*' or '*Hail Mary*' options considered when all else have failed. The primary techniques that fall into this category include:

a. **External, _Non-Invasive_ Cortical Stimulation** – where '*cortical*' (from 'cortex') refers to the *outer* layer of the brain. This option does **_not_** involve any surgery.

The four main techniques that may be used are:

1. *Transcranial Magnetic Stimulation* (TMS).

2. *Repetitive Transcranial Magnetic Stimulation* (rTMS).

3. *Transcranial Direct Current Stimulation* (tDCS).

4. *Electroconvulsive Therapy* (ECT).

With *Transcranial Magnetic Stimulation,* powerful magnetic coils, carefully positioned around a patient's head (but not touching the head itself) are used to generate *pulsating* magnetic fields that stimulate nerves within the brain. In the '*repetitive*' variant, i.e., *rTMS*, the pulsing occurs more often to produce a stronger, longer-lasting effect. TMS was approved by the U.S. FDA, in 2008, as a treatment for depression.

Transcranial Direct Current Stimulation (tDCS) and *Electroconvulsive Therapy* (ECT) both use electrical current, rather than magnetic fields, to stimulate certain parts of the brain. They differ in terms of the current used, tDCS typically using 400 times _LESS_ current than ECT. ECTs, which have to be performed under general anesthetic, intentionally trigger *minor seizures* of the brain. tDCS, on the other hand, does not rely on inducing a seizure. Both these techniques, as with TMS, have often been used to treat chronic, drug-resistant depression. ECTs are sometimes referred to as '*electroshock therapy*'.

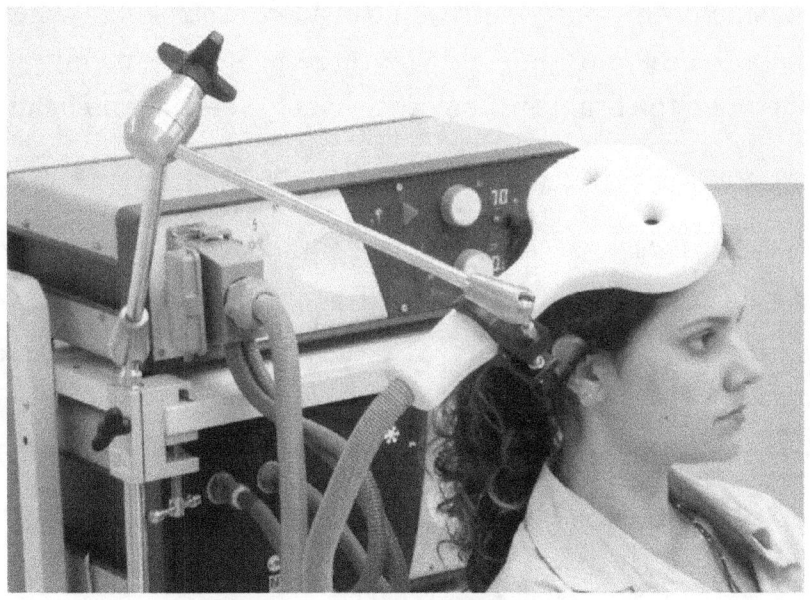

An example of *Transcranial Magnetic Stimulation* (TMS) in use. Note that there is nothing attached to the patient's head.

From Wikipedia, in entry for TMS.

These non-invasive techniques are said to be not as effective in treating CPS as is the invasive option! That probably comes as no surprise to any. Obviously, an invasive procedure, involving the brain, is much more involved, complicated and *consequential.*

b. ___Invasive___, **Brain Stimulation.** There are *two very different techniques* here, though both require <u>openings in the skull</u> to gain access to the brain. With the first technique the electrodes are placed *outside* of the brain, whereas in the second the electrodes are *embedded inside* the brain.

The two techniques are:

1. *Extradural Cortical Stimulation* (ECS).

2. *Deep Brain Stimulation (DBS).*

'*Extradural*' indicates that the procedure is being performed outside of the '*dura mater*', but inside of the skull – where '*dura mater*' is the outermost of the three protective membranes that surround the brain, just below the skull. See diagram below.

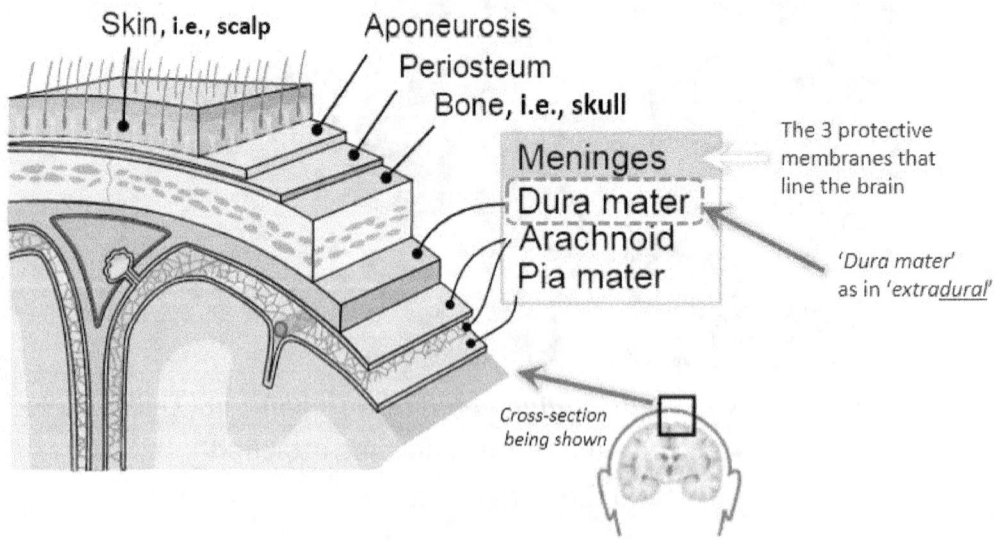

'Dura Mater', as it relates to 'extradural', relative to the skull and the brain.

From Wikipedia.

For *Extradural Cortical Stimulation* one or more openings are made in the skull. Then flat, paddle-like electrodes are strategically placed against the dura mater. Current is applied to the electrodes via an external unit to create the desired brain stimulation.

Extradural Cortical Stimulation is said to be more effective in addressing the symptoms of CPS than the non-invasive techniques. It does not, however, work in all instances. The currently claimed 'success rate' is along the lines of: *'more than 50% of those treated experiencing a greater than 50% decrease in pain'.*

Deep Brain Stimulation takes the invasiveness to the next – and essentially the highest – level when it comes to central nervous system <u>stimulation.</u> With this approach, one or more electrodes, attached to needle-like probes, are inserted deep into the brain – to reach specific targeted areas within the brain. See diagram below.

As with other techniques the stimulation could be provided with an external unit. But, it is not uncommon for the generator (sometimes referred to as a 'brain pace maker') and all the wiring to be implanted inside the patient. This way stimulation can be applied on a long-term basis. This technique is essentially the brain equivalent of *Spinal Cord Stimulation* (SCS).

Deep Brain Stimulation is not a recommended option for treating CPS – though there have been some reports of success. It would typically only be considered in cases where *Extradural Cortical Stimulation* has proved to be effective. At present, this technique, relative to CPS, is most likely to be available, to selected patients, on a tightly-controlled clinical trial basis.

<< Images of *Deep Brain Stimulation* follow >>

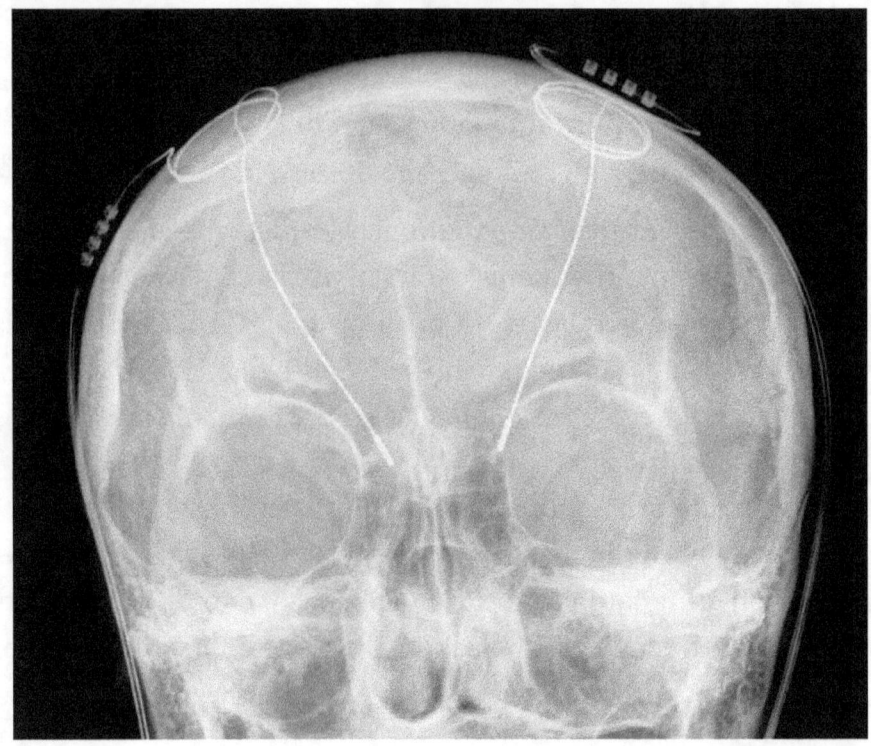

The probes, wiring and electrodes used in
Deep Brain Stimulation as seen in an actual X-Ray.
Note that the probes are placed *deep inside* the brain.

From Wikipedia.

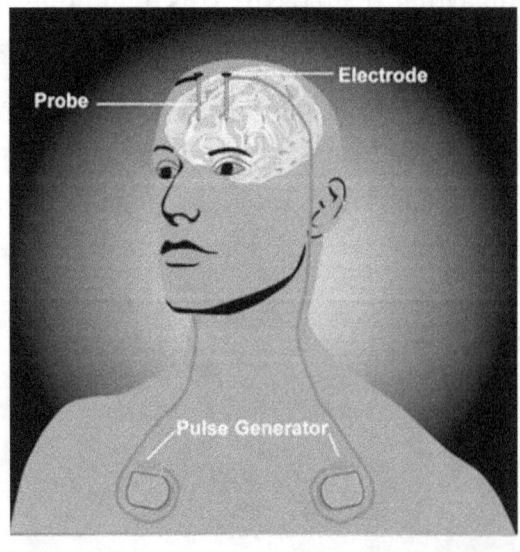

A fully implanted *Deep Brain Stimulation* configuration.

From Wikipedia.

c. Selective *snipping* of specific *nerves* within the brain – so called *Subparietal Leucotomy* – a form of *lobotomy*. Not a recommended option for CPS and only considered in a few, exceptional cases – mainly for clinical research.

d. *Removal* or disabling/*destroying* of specific, targeted portions of the brain – sometimes these portions being as big as golf balls or larger. Ditto, as in 'c' (↑) in terms of applicability.

e. *Cerebrospinal Fluid Injections.* Cerebrospinal Fluid is a *protective* body fluid found around the brain and the spinal column. It serves as both a physical and chemical barrier. Certain pain relief, anesthetic or muscle relaxant medication such as: *Midazolam* (anesthetic/sedative/anti-seizure), *Baclofen* (muscle relaxant) or *Ziconotide* (pain reliever) can be injected directly into the *Cerebrospinal Fluid.* As with all of these treatments, some success has been claimed relative to CPS.

f. A *spinal infusion pump*, often referred to as a *morphine pump* – whereby an implanted pump regularly injects pain medication directly into the spinal column area. The pump will typically contain enough medication to last 1 to 3 months. It can be refilled, fairly easily, using a needle. Morphine pumps are not commonly used in the treatment of CPS, but remain as a 'last resort' option.

WHO SHOULD BE CONSULTED FOR TREATMENT

A primary care doctor, though likely to be the first line of defense, is unlikely to be the best choice for long-term CPS care. In most instances a primary care doctor will persist in referring CPS patients to specialists – well aware that trying to treat CPS is an involved, complicated, and invariably, a thankless process.

If it is an option, consulting a 'good' *pain specialist*, sympathetic to CPS, is obviously the best choice for most sufferers. Seeing a psychiatrist for the psychological aspects of CPS can also be beneficial. Ideally, in a perfect world, the pain specialist and the psychiatrist will coordinate the treatment between them – especially when it comes to the medications being prescribed. However, this may not prove to be as easy or obvious as it sounds. So, it will often fall upon you to do the coordination and tell each of the doctors what you are being prescribed by the other. This lack of coordinated care is a big problem when it comes to CPS. Keep that in mind and always try to see if you can get one doctor to talk to the other – or at a minimum exchange some medical notes.

Given that CPS is indeed a neurological condition seeing a neurologist is another recommended option. Neurologists do understand chronic pain and do know how to try and tackle it at the nerve-level. Depending on the treatment options being considered you may be referred to a *neurosurgeon* (i.e., one that can also do brain surgery).

Some of the other medical professionals that you may opt to consult with should also include: psychologists, therapists and physical therapists.

If you intend to pursue alternate therapies do so with care. There is a concern that chiropractic and deep massage treatments, by being too intense, will just aggravate the hyperalgesia of CPS. *Keep that in mind.* If possible, discuss these alternate approaches with a pain specialist. Doing a lot of Web research and talking to other CPS sufferers, on online forums, can also be beneficial. The last thing you want is something that though well-meaning ends up, unintentionally, making the CPS symptoms worse.

THE PROGNOSIS FOR CPS

The symptoms of CPS will vary and fluctuate, unpredictably, from day-to-day, and sometimes hour-to-hour. There could be periods of tolerable remission – lasting days, maybe longer.

Some treatment options, particularly at the start, may provide considerable relief. However, resistance/tolerance to a given treatment, over time, is known to happen quite often.

Though not that common, CPS is sometimes known to go away, more or less completely, on its own. But, it is best not to hold out hope on this.

There is, as yet, no permanent cure for CPS.

Once you have CPS the chances are that it will be, alas, chronic and lifelong.

CPS is **not** deemed to be life-threatening, nor a condition that noticeably decreases life expectancy.

CPS, however, can be debilitating and can dramatically impact one's quality and enjoyment of life.

The symptoms of CPS are likely to get worse over time due to 3 key reasons: resistance/tolerance to treatments, increase in pain sensitivity (i.e., hyperalgesia) and escalating emotional distress. Suicidal thoughts are often a risk that has to be addressed and monitored.

New treatment options in the future, in particular better drugs (with less side-effects), may offer significant promise down the road. For now, it is best to tackle CPS one day at a time, with always the hope that tomorrow could be another *'good day'*.

DIET

Whether diet can play a realistic role in minimizing the symptoms of CPS has yet to be determined. Given the fickleness of CPS it is unlikely that there is likely to be one particular type of diet that will work across the board. As with so much to do with CPS, any relief via a change in diet is likely to be highly personal. But, it is worth experimenting with different diets on the basis of *'whatever works'* and *'what have you got to lose'*. It is possible that eliminating some food types might help (e.g., raw sugar, lactose, carbs, fats, etc.) Taking Omega-3 and maybe Turmeric might help.

TAKEAWAYS:
CHAPTER 6 – TREATMENT

- ❧ There are a wide range of possible options for treating the main symptoms of CPS ranging from oral medication to brain surgery; with injections, nerve stimulation and non-invasive brain stimulation among the other options.

- ❧ There is no one particular treatment regimen that is considered to be superior to others, with what works well for one unlikely to do so for another – and with always the possibility that what was working well 'last week' might cease to be effective 'next week'.

- ❧ CPS is well known for its (infuriating) *treatment tolerance*; i.e., for the effectiveness of a treatment to diminish over time.

- ❧ Doctors will continue to treat the symptoms, often happy to go along with '*whatever that works*'.

- ❧ There is, as yet, no cure for CPS.

- ❧ Local anesthetics, in particular *Lidocaine* patches, are known to offer varying degrees of relief – as are TENS units.

- ❧ *Antiepileptic/anticonvulsant (e.g., Pregabalin (*Lyrica) & *Gabapentin (*Neurontin)) and *antidepressant (e.g., Duloxetine (*Cymbalta)) medications have had a good track-record in treating CPS.

- ❧ The use of opioids in the context of CPS, in particular long-term usage, remains controversial, vexing and divisive – with it recognized that opioids can worsen the *hyperalgesia* of CPS.

- ❧ If CPS was probably due to a previous injury, typically to the spinal column, it is common to keep on trying to treat that injury.

- ❧ While it is, of course, the invasive technique that is said to be more effective, *non-invasive* brain stimulation, e.g., rTMS, would be worth considering if it is at all an available option.

7.
RESOURCES

If you suffer from Central Pain Syndrome, you are not alone.

At least **3 million people** worldwide suffer from CPS; most likely much more. It is believed that there are over 5 million adults in the U.S. with fibromyalgia – a condition that in some way appears to be related to CPS.

CPS, definitely falls into the category of '*chronic pain*', and 'chronic pain' in the U.S. is now being talked about as an *epidemic* – much more widespread than diabetes, cancer or heart disease! Given the **50 million** (or so) affected, and the inescapable ties to the highly destructive *opioid use epidemic*, chronic pain is finally getting the attention it deserves – along with the much-needed research funding. So, you are also no longer being overlooked or marginalized. Chronic pain is becoming *mainstream* issue (and the associated stigma becoming progressively less so, though there is still a long way to go).

There is an abundance of resources, particularly online (i.e., the Web), that can help you cope with, and deal with, Central Pain Syndrome. Do not feel that you have to suffer alone, in private; in silence. You are part of a large, caring and sharing community and there are many forums and support groups (local and online) that could be of help.

If you are diagnosed with asthma or diabetes, doctors will often urge you to learn as much as you can about these conditions, **on your own**, since that will definitely help you better deal what lies ahead. Many a doctor would tell you, upfront, that they just do not have the time to go through all the various '*in-and-outs*' of these two conditions, or *even all the* possible treatment options! Hence, why they recommend that you learn as much as you can about asthma/diabetes on your own and then discuss aspects that you think are relevant to you on subsequent visits. *Ditto, if not '**ditto emphasized**', when it comes to CPS.*

There is so much to CPS.

CPS is complex, convoluted and confusing.

A pain doctor or neurologist, however committed and well intentioned, will not have the time to discuss '*everything*' and come up with all of the potential *action plans* that may be applicable to YOU. Plus, you may have not had the chance or felt inclined to discuss all of the 'niggling' things that have been bothering you. So, you have to first help yourself – and then take your findings to your doctor (or doctors).

That you are consulting this book is a great start. I have done my best to capture as much of what is relevant, useful and topical. But, there may be more you can find online or by 'talking' with others in your shoes.

SOME USEFUL ORGANIZATIONS

- ❧ CENTRAL PAIN SYNDROME FOUNDATION
  centralpainsyndromefoundation.com

- ❧ American Chronic Pain Association
  theacpa.org

- ❧ National Fibromyalgia & Chronic Pain Association
  www.fmcpaware.org

- ❧ Institute for Chronic Pain
  www.instituteforchronicpain.org

- ❧ American Pain Society
  americanpainsociety.org

ɷ The British Pain Society
www.britishpainsociety.org

ɷ NATIONAL INSTITUTES OF HEALTH
www.nih.gov

> ➤ National Institute of Neurological Disorders and Stroke (NINDS)
> *www.ninds.nih.gov*

> ➤ National Institute of Arthritis and Musculoskeletal and Skin Diseases (NIAMS)
> *www.niams.nih.gov*

> ➤ National Institute of Mental Health (NIMH)
> *www.nimh.nih.gov*

ɷ National Organization for Rare Disorders (NORD)
rarediseases.org

ɷ National Stroke Association
www.stroke.org

ɷ National Multiple Sclerosis Society
www.nationalmssociety.org

ɷ American Epilepsy Society
www.aesnet.org

ɷ 'Body in Mind' – *Research into the role of the brain & mind in chronic pain*
www.bodyinmind.org

ɷ International Association for the Study of Pain
www.iasp-pain.org

SOME USEFUL WEBSITES

❖ *Healthline* at: *www.healthline.com*

❖ *Mayo Clinic* at: *www.mayoclinic.com*

❖ *WebMD* at: *www.webmd.com*

❖ *Wikipedia* at: *en.wikipedia.org*
   < Often a good place to start. Check the references and make sure to confirm anything that seems too good to be true or 'not right'. >

❖ *Pain* (Your Pain Management Resource) at: *pain.com*

❖ *PainScience* at: *www.painscience.com*

❖ *YouTube videos* at: *youtube.com*
   < Search on appropriate keywords such as 'central pain', 'chronic pain', 'pain sensitization', etc. >

❖ *Fibromyalgia Information Foundation* at: *www.myalgia.com*

❖ *Patients Like Me* at: *www.patientslikeme.com*
   < Type in 'central pain syndrome', 'fibromyalgia' or similar in the "Look up Condition" trench below the navigation buttons. >

❖ *Health Message Boards* at: *www.healthboards.com*
   < Use the 'Search' trench at the top, on the header. >

❖ *Support Groups* at: *www.supportgroups.com*
   < Look for 'chronic pain', 'fibromyalgia', etc. under 'groups' in the menu bar at the top. >

HOW TO BEST USE ABOVE RESOURCES

The resources listed, of even just a selected few, should provide you with plenty of *food-for-thought* in terms of insights, real-life experiences and opinions. With luck, you should see a consistency and commonality in what you learn about CPS – even if it is that nothing can be generalized when it comes to CPS, other than that it is 'awful'. And that, as you will by now know, has already been talked about multiple times in this book.

Double-, triple-check everything (between the resources and even this book) – especially if it sounds '*too good to be true*' or is at odds with what you have previously believed. Make sure the information is from reputable, credible sources; e.g., National Institutes/Societies, Mayo Clinic, WebMd, etc. Poke and prod. Make it a fun challenge. Set some goals.

Take notes (which is always a good thing). Go back, look through your notes and create a new list of 'talking points'. Discuss findings with family and friends. You could opt to do so online, albeit *cautiously*. Be aware that if you venture online that you might end up getting various diverse viewpoints, some of it unlikely to be relevant or useful. *Beware* that there could be disguised '*paid content*' (in addition to the obvious advertisements) as well as '*crooks*' eager to sell you snake-oil! Just be careful. Just like chronic pain, online scamming is now an epidemic.

Compare how the treatment options you have received and are currently receiving match up against those mentioned in this book and online. You are bound to find disconnects, contradictions and controversy – particularly when it comes to some of the drugs (in particular opioids) and nerve/brain stimulation techniques. See what makes sense to you. Take notes or print out the relevant extracts. Discuss them with your doctor or find a doctor specializing in an option that interests you; e.g., *Repetitive Transcranial Magnetic Stimulation* (rTMS).

The online resources I have listed here are the ones that met *my personal criteria for credibility*. They are also, in the main, resources I am familiar with and have consulted when writing this book or one of my previous books. But, of course, I <u>cannot vouch</u> for any of the information that you may find – partly because much of it is frequently updated or being added to.

There are plenty of other resources beyond what I have listed. Depending on where you live you may be able to find *local resources* – in some instances groups that you may be able to join. But, in the case of such groups, if possible, ask around to determine if they are 'legit' and are relevant before you decide to attend any meetings.

So, if you want to go further, do a *search* (ideally using *Google*, but most other reputable search engines might suffice) on '*central pain*'. Some of the *initial entries* you are likely to see have probably already been listed above. But, continue down the entries. See if any catch your interest.

But, please, as ever, be careful when 'strolling through' the Web – it can be a dangerous neighborhood. Make sure your computer has adequate '*Internet Security*' safeguards, use a Web browser such as Google with considerable built-in protection, and avoid anything that looks too 'exotic'. *{Smile}*

Do other searches, e.g., '*central pain*', '*chronic pain*', '*central sensitization*', '*fibromyalgia*', etc.

You don't have to stop there. You can, maybe should, continue on to search: symptoms, the drugs that have been prescribed or are being suggested, the treatments you are currently undertaking as well as any that have been put forward as future options.

The more *you can learn*, the more *empowered you will be* when it comes to being able to *decide on **your future***.

8.
COPING
WITH CPS

Central Pain Syndrome 'sucks', and 'sucks' badly. Of that there should be no doubt or debate.

CPS can be overwhelming and all consuming. It weighs on you, constantly, and wears you down, grindingly, on a daily basis. It impacts your day-to-day existence and that of those around you. It infuriates and is discouraging.

But, you have to try and cope *as best as you can* – and that, of course, is easier said, than done.

In the majority of instances, CPS once it sets in tends to be *lifelong* – albeit with variations in symptoms and *intensity*, fickle periods of *remission,* and times when a treatment option succeeds in making the pain *bearable.*

There is, as yet, no cure for CPS. It, as such, falls into the category of an *incurable condition.* One has to, at some point, *come to terms with that* – however hard that might be.

Though incurable, CPS is **not** life-threatening or deemed to reduce life-expectancy (though some will disagree, while others would not see that as a true blessing). Notwithstanding, CPS causes enormous *emotional distress* – and a heightened incidence of suicidal and self-harm inclinations are a common danger. Perversely, some of the *antidepressants* that have proved to be rather effective in treating CPS, e.g., *Duloxetine* (Cymbalta), are known to aggravate this tendency!

There is, as discussed in chapter 4, *Pain & The Brain*, a large psychological (i.e., mind/brain-related) element to CPS. The more emotionally distressed you are, the less chance you have of '*controlling*' CPS. *The more you get upset about having CPS, the worse the CPS will become!*

It is, indeed, a wicked, vicious-cycle.

Ignoring *mind over matter* altogether, it still has to be acknowledged that a 'healthy' mental attitude towards CPS definitely has to help – if nothing else by slowing down the '*hyperalgesia ↔ emotional distress*' loop. And coping with CPS boils down to <u>trying</u> (as best as you can) to be *realistic* and '*philosophical*' about it, however hard that may be.

Two other appropriate words would be: *resigned* and *stoic*. Being realistically *sanguine* is another way to look at it. But, it is *understood* and appreciated that this is not easy – with the crushing weight of CPS bearing down on you, relentlessly. This, as will be discussed further, is not being negative, defeatist or 'giving into CPS'. It is actually you standing up to CPS and proclaiming, categorically: '*Enough, is enough. I am not going to let CPS ruin my life any further. This is it. I am not going to let CPS grind me down.*' Yes, it is not going to be easy. But, it is your BEST hope.

{This is meant to be a 'Self Help' book and as such all of this is meant to help you, not to annoy you! Be patient. At this stage, what have you got to lose? {Smile}}

THE DENIAL HAS TO STOP AT SOME POINT

It appears to be the norm that *accepting* the *incurability* of CPS is a huge challenge.

Others have enormous trouble accepting that *they have* CPS to begin with – never mind its incurability.

Thus, it is not uncommon for those suffering from CPS to be in denial for a very, very long time – even for years.

There appears to be 4 major reasons for this inclination towards denial:

1. Indications by doctors that they will eventually find a cure for the pain as long as they keep on trying different things (and you continue to be patient and tolerant). In some instances doctors will be **reluctant to admit** that the pain is due to CPS, rather than from a treatable injury or inflammation -- and as such is going to be hard to remedy. *(Refer to chapter 5 where there is a section on this 'reluctance'.)*

2. Perception that CPS, despite the ongoing, long-term pain, just does not seem that serious an illness compared to other conditions (say MS or diabetes), and as such should go away in time.

3. Belief that it, despite its searing severity, is still 'only pain' and as such somebody, somewhere must have a magic, silver-bullet treatment that can make that pain go away.

4. That accepting CPS indicates that: one is giving 'into the pain', is signaling an unwillingness to keep on fighting *the battle*, and, in general, succumbing to 'negative' thoughts – when one is striving to be positive at all times.

First and foremost, if you are suffering from CPS you have the **RIGHT** to be in denial. It is the least of the consolations you can enjoy.

But, at some point, maybe after a few years (*say 4 to 5 years*), you need to CONFRONT CPS, head on.

The 4 -5 years is not arbitrary and definitely **not** meant to be facetious. Some of you are going to need that long, but, hopefully, not much more than that. IF you can do it sooner, so much the better. But, as with all things CPS, it should be – and it will be – '*whatever works for YOU*'.

It is going to take time before you are ready to accept that you really do have CPS, that CPS really sucks, and, in all reality, you are going to have CPS for the remainder of your life.

It is a HUGE step, but one you have to eventually make.

Among its many annoying traits, CPS does play tricks on your perception of time. You get so preoccupied living with, and dealing with, CPS that you lose sight of time. That is 'OK'. Par for the course. It also means time can move on without you getting around to doing things that you want to do. That is why the 4 – 5 years is not unreasonable.

There will be a lot going on at the beginning. It could already be 'years' before you realize or are told you have CPS. That is a pity – nonetheless, yet another reality of suffering from CPS. But, once you know you have CPS there is still much that has to be done – up front.

To begin with, you probably will be anxious to find out WHY and HOW CPS set in. Getting to the bottom of that will take time.

Then there are the treatment options. Everything will take time. Doctors are not in a hurry. They do not have CPS, YOU do. They don't, despite any and all of their platitudes, share your urgency. They will want to 'go slow' with the medications. They will want several months of 'med. checks'. They will want to perform exploratory procedures, get more MRIs. Time, inexorably, will move on. Before you realize it, 4-months have gone … half a year … then a year. So on, and so forth. A couple of years later the doctors will still be trying out different medications or processes. You continue living with CPS, constantly battling the pain and wondering if there ever will be an end to this 'living hell'. If you are paying for the treatment, or even some of it, the costs could be horrendous!

In time, notwithstanding hope-against-hope, you will slowly come to realize that CPS is very real – and that it is here to stay. This is when you need to start thinking about confronting the denial.

Finally accepting that you have CPS and that CPS, as yet, is incurable is NOT admitting defeat, or being negative! To think this might be so, is to be unrealistic and not fair on yourself.

Reality is neither positive nor negative. Reality is reality; reality is what it is – **reality is life**. Reality is what life is going to be. Reality is not easy, but reality is what you have to live with.

That CPS is currently incurable sucks. But, CPS is far from being alone on that count. There are many other incurable conditions. While some will contend that some of the other 'incurables' are not as painful or debilitating as CPS, it is also the case that there are conditions/situations that are worse – far worse.

CPS is a pain, quite literally, BUT it is not life threating or one that is believed to effect life expectancy. *Yes, it is, nonetheless, life limiting in terms of quality of life.* However, it could be much worse. And that is what YOU have to (please) consider. Despite the pain and the anguish, you have to look around. There are others in worse shape, possibly more pain. Yes, of course, that doesn't help you with your pain, but can you, at least, see that you are not alone – and that incurable pain and suffering is *NOT* limited to CPS.

This is the step you have to make ... the threshold you have to cross ... the bridge you have to put behind you.

You, at some point, have to stop the denial and slowly, but surely, accept the unpleasant reality of CPS.

You can't start coping with CPS, until you finally get around to accepting that you have CPS – and that CPS is said to be incurable.

Yes, of course, there is a possibility that by some miracle you could wake up tomorrow and discover the pain of CPS has gone – and it is never to come back. Miracles do happen – though not often. *You can always hope for the miracle while, grudgingly, accepting the reality.* That is OK. That is also your right. Let's hope you are indeed one of the lucky few that miraculously experience a complete reversal of CPS – however, in the meantime you should steel yourself to bravely confront the stark realities of CPS.

GO THROUGH THE GRIEVING PROCESS

Since way back in 1985, the guiding principle of my life has been:

"If you lose all your wealth, you have lost nothing.
If you lose your health, you have lost something.
But, if you lose your credibility you have lost everything."

In the context of CPS, the second line applies – in full. If you have CPS, your health has been undermined and you have, indeed, *lost something in life.*

This loss is real and nobody who understands CPS will ever question you on that.

If you have CPS you should consider going through the grieving process once you realize you are ready, *at last*, to go beyond denial.

Yes, as it happens 'denial and isolation' is the FIRST stage of the *'Grief & Loss'* process. So, this dovetails in nicely.

I am NOT going to talk about the grieving process here – because many of you may have your own *interpretation of it*. It is a well-known topic and it is easy enough to find plenty of information about it locally (e.g., a library or doctor's office) or online. There should also be plenty of people who will be happy to talk to you about it.

The bottom line here, however, is that you really should consider going through the grieving/loss process, in its entirety, in the context of CPS.

Get angry. Rail against CPS. Curse CPS. Rue the day you heard about CPS. Rant and rave. You have the RIGHT to be angry, very angry. CPS sucks.

Feel sorry for yourself. You sure have the right do be so. CPS sure sucks. Take your time. It is not fair – but, life often never is. Yes, ask yourself, more than once: *'why me?'*. **'Why ME?'** 'Why ME?' Then, just spare a thought. It could be worse; it could be much worse. Yes, it could. Don't delude yourself. CPS sucks, but there are other conditions that suck worse.

Life is never black or white. Life is all about a spectrum of grays. Though you may have never thought about it as such, life is all about compromises. And living and coping with CPS is one of those compromises. Do not think of it as you having been compromised, think of it as a compromise you have to now deal with.

Yes. Yes. Yes. All of this is so much easier to say than do. That is understood. Nonetheless, it has to be said, so that you get the chance to consider *the following suggestion*.

> Yes. A suggestion for YOU,
> *which is as follows.*

That is what this chapter is all about. *Suggestions ... recommendations ... self-help guidelines* – given that this is indeed a 'self-help' book.

It is your CPS, your life ... your right!

Nobody can, and should, tell you how YOU should try to deal with YOUR CPS. It is YOUR CPS and only you, and you alone, can determine how you want to deal with it. That is understood. That is a given.

So, it is over to you, but with the urging that you should consider what is being said in this chapter.

The ball is, however, in your court. YOU have to decide what you are going to do with 'that ball'. *{So please read on.}*

THE BOTTOM LINE

Given the 'chiseled in stone', *pain-brain connection* (per chapter 4), we have to accept, whether we like it or not, that the brain plays a critical role when it comes to CPS. That is reality – and we are now at the stage where we have to continually confront reality.

To avoid all misunderstandings and incredulity, lets, as we did earlier, take 'mind over matter' off the table – i.e., the expectations that the misery of CPS can be kept in check just via mind 'control'. That is unrealistic for most.

'Mind over matter', at a minimum, requires a mental discipline that takes years of hard work to acquire, unusual mental agility, and lots of luck. All that said, if you are interested in exploring it, it is indeed a worthwhile and rewarding objective. Meditation (in particular 'brain meditation') and yoga are the best ways to start. That is all we are going to say about 'mind over matter'.

Once you have finally got around to accepting you have CPS, you need to, in essence, make your peace with CPS. This is yet another degree, another level, of acceptance. Making the peace could take some time too. It is another process. *This is when you agree, with yourself, that you are no longer going to rail against CPS.*

You are going to accept the misery of CPS as a given. Something you have to live with every day. Yes, it sucks, BUT you have fought it for long enough – and YOU, better than anyone else, knows that fighting CPS hasn't done you any favors.

Again, this is not to say you are giving up hope. You keep hope alive, always – you just stop fighting CPS and thinking of CPS as your enemy. Of course, CPS is not your friend. Getting CPS is one of the worst things that has ever happened to you. But, now you have to live with it, day-to-day, and fighting CPS just makes it WORSE!

What we are trying to achieve is some amount of MENTAL PEACE.

A reduction in the anguish, the turmoil, the anger, the anxiety.

Yes, easier said than done.

Every new degree, every iota, of mental peace you can gain will help you – help you feel better. The pain will **not** go away. It will, however, not get you down to the same level as before. Yes, it is an extension of that old mantra about being '*always positive*'.

What have YOU got to lose, at this stage? If anything, there is much you can gain in terms of a slightly better quality of life. Slightly better is better than none. Yes, you have to do it in increments. Baby steps. But, each step will count.

> Once you have made peace with CPS you need to make peace with YOURSELF.

You need to practice some form of meditation on a daily basis – ideally multiple times a day. You have to, by hook or by crook, start gaining some degree of control over your brain – your mind, your thoughts, your inner psyche. Yes, CPS would have done a 'job' on your mind and brain. Now is when YOU set out to push back on that. Regain some of what you have lost. It can be done. Yes, it will be hard, but it should not be impossible.

Patience and perseverance every day, 7-days a week.

Meditate. Do yoga. Go for long walks. Do whatever exercises that you can manage. All of these activities trigger 'good' chemicals to be activated within your brain.

Talk to your brain. Discuss CPS with your brain. Always aspire to find peace with yourself. Calm your mind.

By now you know your CPS better than anybody.

IF you haven't already figured it out, set about determining YOUR exact CPS related symptoms, i.e., which pains and sensations **MUST be due to CPS** and which ones can be tied, definitely, to a genuine injury or inflammation. You have to do this. Nobody else can. By now you must know what is what. Working this out is key.

If you really are not sure, then you must have a long, candid discussion with your pain doctor. <u>*DEMAND truthfulness*</u>, facts and accuracy. Make it clear you are no longer interested in being 'humored'. Insist that you are told as to which symptoms are suspected of being CPS-related. If your doctor is still vague it might be time to find another!

Once you have determined the CPS related symptoms, really, really, really spend a lot of time, on your own, with your mind, understanding what it is all about. *IF a symptom is CPS-related YOU know by now that 'it' can only be addressed at the central nervous system level.* So, go back and work out if that is happening in terms of your current treatment plan. Recall the treatments you have had in the past. Where they aimed at the CNS? Be realistic about CPS and the treatment you are getting. IF a pain is CPS-related you are not going to make it better by getting treatment for a non-existing inflammation or injury.

So, in the end, it is you and your CPS.

You have to help yourself. Finding peace with yourself will certainly help – and that is *doable*. Every bit of mental peace you can muster will help you. It will make life more tolerable. So, this has to be your new goal. Pushing ahead, every day, to soothe the mind to help the CPS.

That concludes the self-help oriented suggestion spiel. *{SMILE}*

I wish you all the best.

৭০ ෴ ෴ ෴

GLOSSARY & MAIN ACRONYMS

'-*ALGIA*': Latin for pain and suffering; found in terms such as my*algia* (muscle pain) & fibromy*algia* (tissue/muscle pain).

ALLODYNIA: Pain from things that should not normally be painful, e.g., touch or feel of clothing.

ANALGESIC: A painkiller; any medication to achieve *analgesia*, i.e., to be without pain.

ANESTHESIA: Medicine to temporarily reduce the sensation or awareness of pain via blocking pain signals, relaxing muscles or inducing memory loss.

ANEURYSM: A weakness in a blood vessel that results in a localized, balloon-like bulge of blood.

ANTIARRHYTHMIC: Abnormal heart rhythms.

ARACHNOIDITIS: Painful inflammation of the '*arachnoid*' -- the middle layer of the protective '*meninges*' – that can cause neurological complications.

ARTERIOVENOUS MALFORMATION (AVM): Often a congenital condition where an abnormal, vulnerable-to-rupture, connection exists between arteries and veins in the brain.

ARTHRITIS: Painful inflammation and stiffness in one or more body joints.

ATAXIA: Difficulty coordinating and controlling body movements.

AUTONOMIC NERVES: Nerves that make up the *autonomic nervous system* and connect the heart, lungs, stomach, bladder, etc. to the spinal cord.

AUTONOMIC NERVOUS SYSTEM (ANS): Part of the *peripheral nervous system* responsible for the functioning of vital internal organs such as the heart, lungs, stomach, intestines, bladder, genitalia, etc.

AUTONOMIC: The involuntary, but vital, functions performed by the body, such as that of maintaining breathing, heart rate, digestion, etc., to keep a body alive.

BRAIN CENTRAL PAIN (BCP): Now considered to be Central Pain Syndrome – even if it is post-stroke related.

BRAIN: The most important organ in the human body.

BRAIN STEM: A part of the brain, towards its rear, that connects the rest of the brain with the spinal cord.

CAUDA EQUINA SYNDROME: Damage to spinal nerves at the end of the *spinal cord*, the so called "horse's tail" (i.e., cauda equine) that can result in serious complications in body parts around the pelvic area.

CENTRAL NERVES: Nerves in the brain and the spinal cord; i.e., part of the CNS.

CENTRAL NERVOUS SYSTEM (CNS): Brain, brain stem and spinal cord.

CENTRAL PAIN SYNDROME (CPS): Nervous system-related condition caused by damage or dysfunction of the central nervous system.

CENTRAL PAIN: Pain associated with the central nervous system.

CENTRAL SENSITIZATION: The central nervous system becoming conditioned over time, due to persistent pain, to be more sensitive, severe and reactive to all pain.

CEREBELLUM: Latin for '*little brain*', it is the brain component that is key to controlling movement, which is made up of two hemispheres, situated behind the brain stem and, as such, below the main, bigger part of the brain (i.e., the *cerebrum*).

CEREBROSPINAL: Having to do with the brain and spine.

CEREBRUM: The main part of the brain (made up of two hemispheres), which is responsible for many of the functions performed by the brain.

CHARCOT-MARIE-TOOTH DISEASE (CMT): A group of inherited disorders of the *peripheral nervous system* that result in nerve damage in the arms and legs. Also known as 'Hereditary Motor and Sensory Neuropathy' (HMSN) or 'Peroneal Muscular Atrophy'.

CHOREOATHETOSIS: Involuntary, irregular twisting and writhing.

CHRONIC PAIN: Pain that has lasted, unabated, for more than 4-6 months and may have morphed during that time to include the symptoms of CPS.

CHRONIC: Any condition that persists for more than a few months or recurs, consistently.

CNS: Central Nervous System.

COMPLEX REGIONAL PAIN SYNDROME (CRPS): See '*Reflex Sympathetic Dystrophy Syndrome*'.

CONVULSIVE: Having to do with convulsions – spasms.

CORD CENTRAL PAIN (CCP): Now Central Pain Syndrome – where the 'cord' refers to the spinal cord.

CORTICAL: Outer layer of an organ, e.g., brain. From '*cortex*'.

CORTICOSTEROIDS (CORTICOIDS): In the context of pain, refers to synthetic steroids that imitate the natural hormones produced by the adrenal glands.

CPS: Central Pain Syndrome.

CRANIAL NERVES: Nerves that are directly connected to the brain, rather than the spinal cord, and include those responsible for vision, eye movement, smell, hearing, balance, taste, head movement, etc.

CUTANEOUS: Having to do with the skin.

DÉJERINE-ROUSSY SYNDROME Now Central Pain Syndrome; Déjerine & Roussy were two French neurologists.

DIABETES: A group of diseases having to do with too much 'blood sugar' (*blood glucose*) in the bloodstream.

DURA MATTER/DURAL: Outermost of the three protective membranes (the *meninges*) that sheath the brain and spinal cord.

DYSESTHESIA: Abnormal sensation of touch due to a neurological condition.

EDEMA: Swelling due to injury or inflammation.

ELECTROCONVULSIVE THERAPY (ECT): Once known as '*electroshock therapy*' or '*shock treatment*', the process of trying to treat mental disorders by electrically inducing seizures under anesthesia.

ENCEPHALITIS: Acute inflammation of the brain – typically due to a virus.

ENDOGENOUS: Produced or originating within a living thing.

ENDORPHINS: The body's naturally occurring pain reducing opioid-like hormones.

EPIDURAL: On or around the outside of the *dura matter* layer of the meninges – typically in the context of the spinal cord.

EPILEPSY: Recurrent seizures due to neurological disorders in the brain.

EXTRADURAL: Same as '*epidural*', but used more often in the context of the brain as opposed to the spinal cord.

FACET JOINT: Joints in the spine that in addition to providing the flexibility for the upper body to bend and twist serve as the openings through which the *spinal nerves* emerge from within the *vertebral column*.

FIBROMYALGIA: A chronic condition, more common among women, resulting in widespread pain and tenderness, coupled with fatigue and emotional distress.

GUILLAIN–BARRÉ SYNDROME (GBS): A disorder where the body's immune system attacks nerve cells in the *peripheral nervous system* – as such the peripheral nervous system equivalent to *Multiple Sclerosis* which is when the attacked nerves are part of the *central nervous system* (CNS).

HEMICHOREOATHETOSIS: '*Choreoathetosis*' just on one side of the body.

HEMIHYPESTHESIA: '*Hypesthesia*' restricted to just one side of the body.

HYPERALGESIA: Heightened sensitivity to pain.

HYPERPATHIA: A variant of hyperalgesia also having to do with pain exaggeration due to a neurological disorder.

HYPERSENSITIVITY: Excessive, beyond normal, sensitivity.

HYPESTHESIA/HYPOESTHESIA: Partial loss of sensitivity to physical sensation, e.g., touch.

HYPOTHALAMUS: From the Greek for 'under *thalamus*', this being the part of the brain responsible for controlling how the nervous system gets access to the body's hormones.

IATROGENIC: Unintended (negative) consequences from medical attention/treatment.

INFRACTION: A violation or infringement of a 'system'.

LACERATING: To roughly tear or cut deeply.

LEPROSY: A bacterial disease, transmitted through droplets from sneezing or coughing, which can cause extensive skin and nerve damage – though it is now curable with long-term drugs.

LEUCOTOMY: Surgical removal of nerve fibers within the brain – once used as a means of treating mental illness.

LOBOTOMY: Another term for '*Leucotomy*'.

LUMBAR PUNCTURE: Another term for '*Spinal Tap*'.

LYME DISEASE: A bacterial infection, primarily transmitted by ticks – named, in 1975, after a town in Connecticut (U.S.) where the disease was first identified for what it was.

MALARIA: A parasitic, blood-infection carried by mosquitos which can be serious, even life threating, without proper treatment.

MENINGES: The three protective membranes that sheath the brain and the spinal cord.

MERALGIA PARESTHETICA: Pinching of a nerve to the thigh resulting in pain, tingling and numbness of that area.

MIND OVER MATTER: Leveraging the power of the mind (or brain) to prevail over physical challenges.

MONONEUROPATHY: Nerve disorder just affecting one nerve.

MORPHINE: A powerful, addictive, pain relieving drug derived from the opium poppy.

MOTOR NEUROPATHY: Nerve disorder involving nerves associated with movement.

MS: Multiple Sclerosis.

MULTIPLE SCLEROSIS (MS): A nervous system-related disease, believed to be caused by a malfunction to the autoimmune system, where the insulation that protects nerves are attacked and damaged by the body's immune system.

MYELITIS: Inflammation of the spinal cord.

MYELOMALACIA: Softening of the spinal cord.

MYOFASCIAL (PAIN): Having to do with muscle (or soft tissue) pain.

NARCOTIC: Any pain reducing *opioid*.

NERVOUS SYSTEM: Consists of the CNS, sensory organs (such as the eyes and ears) and all the interconnecting nerves.

NEURAL: Having to do with nerves or the nervous system.

NEURALGIA: A sharp, stabbing pain or burning sensation caused by nerve damage.

NEUROFIBROMATOSIS: Inherited disorder that results in tumors to form in the brain, spinal cord and nerves.

NEUROLOGICAL: Having to do with the nervous system.

NEUROLOGIST: A doctor specializing in nervous system & central nervous system disorders (including the brain).

NEUROPATHIC (PAIN): Pain that results from injury or malfunction to the body's nervous system, be it the central or peripheral nervous system. CPS falls into this category. Opposite of '*nociceptive pain*'.

NEUROPATHY: Problems having to do with nerves, whether it be pain, weakness, numbness, etc.

NOCICEPTIVE (PAIN): Pain caused by an actual stimulation of nerve cells and includes pain due to: cuts, burns, sprains, inflammation, bumps, etc. Related to '*nociceptors*'. Opposite of '*neuropathic pain*'.

NOCICEPTORS: Sensory nerve cells within the body that are responsible for informing the CNS whenever they detect anything that could harm the body.

NONSTEROIDAL: Not having to do with *steroids*.

OPIOID: Meaning '*opium like*', and applying to any substance, natural or synthetic, that has the characteristics of *opium*.

OPIUM: Strong, addictive drug, known for its pain-relieving properties, extracted from the '*opium poppy seed*'.

OSTEOARTHRITIS: Arthritis due to '*wear and tear*' to tissue around bones caused by aging, injury or obesity; sometimes referred to as '*degenerative joint disease*'.

PARKINSON'S DISEASE: Progressive disorder of the *central nervous system* that affects movement and can often cause tremors.

PERCEPTION: Recognition and registration by the brain of a *sensory 'signal'* (a '*sensation*').

PERIPHERAL NERVOUS SYSTEM: Nervous system outside of the CNS.

PITUITARY GLAND: Pea-sized gland located at the base of the brain that produces key hormones that control much of what happens in the body – so much so that it is called the '*master gland*'.

PLACEBO: A substance with no active medical or therapeutic properties used (in clinical tests) in place of the '*real thing*' – with the name being Latin for '*I shall please*'.

POLIO: Full name, *poliomyelitis*, is a highly contagious, but preventable, viral disease, which mainly affects young children, that compromises the central nervous system and leads to paralysis.

POLYNEUROPATHY: Nerve disorder involving multiple nerves.

POSTERIOR MYELITIS: Inflammation of the spinal cord (*myelitis*) restricted just to the backside of the cord.

PRION DISORDERS/DISEASES: Also, known as '*Transmissible Spongiform Encephalopathies*' (TSEs) are a group of infectious, but rare, conditions that progressively affect the nervous system.

PRURITUS: Itching – and the desire to scratch.

PSYCHOLOGICAL: Having to do with the mind, and as such pertaining to the mental and emotional state of a person.

REFLEX SYMPATHETIC DYSTROPHY (RSD) SYNDROME: Also, known as '*Complex Regional Pain Syndrome*' (CRPS), has many similarities to '*Central Pain*' in that it results in chronic arm or leg pain following an injury, stroke, surgery or heart attack.

RHEUMATIC: Having to do with joints, muscle and soft tissue.

RHIZOTOMY: Surgical procedure to 'shut off' nerves by severing nerve roots in the spinal cord.

SACROILIAC JOINT: Two joints, on either side of the pelvis, the sciatic nerves passing very close to them.

SENSATION: In this context, it has to do with sensory impulses transmitted to the brain.

SENSORIMOTOR NEUROPATHY: Nerve disorder involving nerves having to do with feeling (i.e., sensory) as well as movement (i.e., motor).

SENSORY NEUROPATHY: Nerve disorder involving nerves that provide feeling.

SHINGLES: A viral infection that causes a painful skin rash, and can result in long-term nerve pain, that arises due to the body, for reasons as yet unknown, reactivating the previously dormant chickenpox virus. Also, known as '*Herpes Zoster*'.

SPASM: Involuntary muscle contractions.

SPASTICITY: Muscle stiffness and muscle spasms.

SPINAL CANAL: Cavity contained within the vertebrae to house the spinal cord.

SPINAL COLUMN: Another word for '*spine*' and '*vertebral column*'.

SPINAL CORD: A thin, ~18" long tube of nervous tissue and support/protective cells that runs from the bottom of the skull to the lumbar region – enclosed within the vertebral column.

SPINAL DISC: Rubbery protective discs between each pair of vertebrae that act as shock absorbers, facilitate spine mobility and helps hold up the spine.

SPINAL FUSION: A major surgery to create a 'bridge' between adjoining vertebrae by means of a bone graft.

SPINAL NERVES: 31-pairs of nerves, connected to the spinal cord, emerging from either side of the vertebral column, that carry nerve signals to do with the senses, movement and bodily functions between the spinal cord and the rest of the body.

SPINAL TAP: Withdrawal of fluid from the lower part of the spinal canal using a needle. Also, known '*Lumbar Puncture*'.

SPINE: Another name for *backbone* and the *vertebral column*.

STENOSIS: The abnormal narrowing (i.e., constriction) of a pathway; e.g., the spinal canal.

STEROID: Natural and synthetic chemicals; the natural ones, made by the body, are usually hormones that help organs, tissues and cells function as they should.

STROKE: Brain damage due to a disruption to the blood vessels serving the brain.

SUBPARIETAL LEUCOTOMY: Leucotomy performed inside the brain.

SYNDROME: When a combination of symptoms is associated with, or defines, a particular condition.

SYRINGOMYELIA: A harmful cyst within the spinal cord.

TETHERED CORD SYNDROME: Neurological disorder caused by tissue attachments within the spinal column hampering the movement of the spinal cord.

THALAMIC (PAIN) SYNDROME: Now, Central Pain Syndrome.

THALAMUS (THALAMIC): A part of the brain, right in the middle, that acts like a 'router' -- processing and routing sensory information around the brain.

TRANSCRANIAL: Through the skull (a.k.a. *cranium*).

TRANSCUTANEOUS: *'Cutaneous'* refers to the skin and *'trans-'* to 'across' – so this denotes across or through the skin.

TRANSDERMAL: Delivery of medication through the skin; *'dermal'* referring to skin as in dermatologist.

TRANSVERSE MYELITIS: Inflammation on both sides of the spinal cord (*myelitis*).

TUBERCULOSIS (TB): Infectious bacterial disease that mainly attacks the lungs but can also affect other parts of the body.

VASCULAR: Related to vessels, in particular blood vessels.

VERTEBRA: The small bones that together make up the backbone (a.k.a. spine, vertebral column).

VERTEBRAL COLUMN: ~33 small bones, i.e., the vertebra, separated by spinal discs, that together make up the human backbone (a.k.a. spine).

INDEX

46, 49, 82, 93, 114, 115 – 118,
120 - 122

Spinal Cord Stimulation 82, 93

Spinal Disc 33 -34, 40, 78, 121 - 122

Spinal Nerves 33 – 34, 78 – 79, 115,
117, 121

Spinal Surgery 67

Spinal Tap See '*Lumbar Puncture*'

Spine See '*Spinal Column*'

Stiffness 18, 22, 37, 114, 120

Stroke 6, 18, 23 – 26, 36, 40, 42, 70
– 71, 101, 115, 120 – 121

Suicidal 88, 97, 105

TAKEAWAYS 16, 22, 42, 65, 74, 98

TENS Units 75, 77, 80 – 81, 98

Touch 2, 6, 15, 29, 39, 63, 114, 116
– 117

Transcranial Magnetic Stimulation
((r)TMS) 90 – 91, 103, 121

Tuberculosis 24, 42, 122

Tumors 6, 23, 28, 30, 34, 36, 41 –
42, 66, 118

Vertebra 23, 32 – 34, 67, 117, 120 –
122

Vertebral Column See '*Spinal
Column*'

Yoga 54, 56, 63, 65, 83, 111, 113

Quick Guide To
Brain Meditation

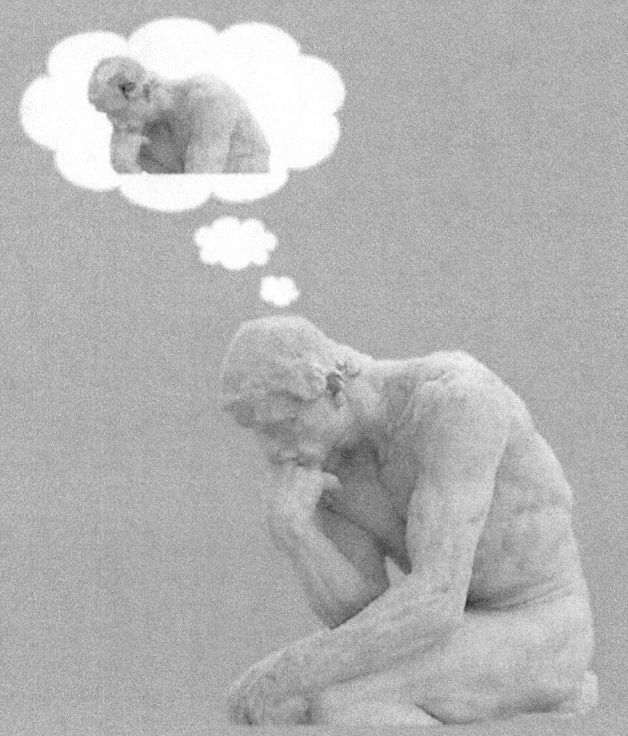

Anura Guruge

www.ingramcontent.com/pod-product-compliance
Lightning Source LLC
Chambersburg PA
CBHW080256180526

45167CB00006B/2553